# CHRISTOPHER NORWOOD

ALSO BY CHRISTOPHER NORWOOD

*About Paterson:*
*The Making and Unmaking of an American City*

# AT
# HIGHEST
# RISK

# AT
# HIGHEST
# RISK

Environmental Hazards to
Young and Unborn Children

McGRAW-HILL BOOK COMPANY

NEW YORK    ST. LOUIS    SAN FRANCISCO
MEXICO    DÜSSELDORF    TORONTO

Excerpt from John Pilger's article "The Gook Hunter"
© 1979 by The New York Times Company.
Reprinted by permission.

Lines from Robert Graves' poem "Warning to Children"
are reprinted by permission of Curtis Brown, Ltd.;
copyright © 1929 by Robert Graves, renewed 1957.

2 3 4 5 6 7 8 9 B P B P 8 7 6 5 4 3 2 1 0

LIBRARY OF CONGRESS CATALOGING IN PUBLICATION DATA
Norwood, Christopher.
   At highest risk.
   Includes index.
   1. Environmentally induced diseases in children.
2. Abnormalities, Human—Etiology.   I. Title.
RJ383.N67      618.9'2      79-20053
ISBN 0-07-047453-2

Book design by Earl Tidwell.

TO THE MEMORY OF PETER B. ARDERY

# CONTENTS

# ACKNOWLEDGMENTS

This book began, although I did not know it then, with a little boy named Binkie who used to live on my block in New York City. Once when I was delivering block association newsletters, he helped me for quite a while. Eventually I asked him if he didn't want to quit and go play, but he shook his head. "It's good to help your neighbor," he said with great determination. Of course, I was irrevocably charmed, but I later learned this helpful child could also be so troublesome that three second-grade teachers had already refused to have him in their classes. His strange swings between charm and uncontrollable anger did not seem to be readily explainable. As more press accounts began to appear about behavior changes caused by food additives and about brain injury from low levels of lead absorption, I wondered whether environmental carelessness might somehow explain a child like Binkie—a child who clearly thought that the good lay in helping his neighbors, but who was too socially destructive to get through second grade. I don't know the answer in his individual case; but it is now becoming obvious that environmental carelessness has reached a level where it explains many children much like Binkie.

This book is a relentless exposition of problems. I would like to qualify it with the idea that we are too often outraged by the minor inconveniences and accidents which technology may inflict on us from time to time. In a world as complex as ours, there are bound to be occasional lapses. Accidents will happen. We should be more tolerant of the proverbial—or literal—mouse that gets trapped in the loaf of bread on the assembly line and save our anger to fight the serious hazards and pollutants that are a mass threat.

I also want to say a few words in defense of the beleaguered government scientist and even the beleaguered government bureaucrat. When I was writing this book, people would very often ask me if the subject matter was not very depressing. Actually, I was less depressed about our environmental prospects when I completed the book than when I had begun it. One reason for this is that doing the research taught me we have some very good and concerned health specialists working in our government. Their advice may not always be followed at the moment that environmental decisions are made—such decisions are often more political than scientific in nature—but their presence is certainly a base from which to work for improvement. It is not my belief that our environmental dilemmas are hopeless or insoluble.

I want to thank the New York Public Library for the use of the Frederick Lewis Allen Room and the helpful and charming staff of the New York Academy of Medicine Library, particularly Bill Landers, Donald Simmons, Linda O'Callaghan, Ada Gams, and Carl Hodo, for their constant assistance.

Dr. Robert W. Miller, Dr. Howard Ulfelder, Dr. Jerry Rice, Professor Vilma Hunt, Dr. Samuel Shapiro, Dr. Robert Kapp, Dr. Jane Lin-Fu, Ruth Lubic, R.N., Dr. Charlotte Silverman, and Dr. Robert Albrecht had the great kindness to read portions of this manuscript. I thank them for their helpful comments, their incisive thoughts, and their time. Any errors are, of course, my own.

I also thank the many people I interviewed in the course of writing this book for the time they spent with me. The American medical community and research community are, on the whole, notably generous in explaining their work.

For support in times of need I thank: John H. Norwood, Jr., Ralph Harris, Martin Stansfeld, Forrest Hoover, Hamilton Hoover, Sanford Schwartz, my dear editor Peggy Tsukahira—and my friends Elizabeth Cramer and Susan Previant Lee.

C.N.

Children, if you dare to think
Of the greatness, rareness, muchness,
Fewness of this precious only
Endless world in which you say
You live, you think of things like this:
Blocks of slate enclosing dappled
Red and green, enclosing tawny
Yellow nets, enclosing white
And black acres of dominoes,
Where a neat brown paper parcel
Tempts you to untie the string.

ROBERT GRAVES
*"Warning to Children"*

# Chapter 1

# A BIG PROBLEM FOR LITTLE PEOPLE

The time has come to consider the effect of an increasingly toxic environment on the health of the young and unborn. It has long been recognized that immature organisms, especially in the womb, are acutely sensitive to agents of disease. This is true for biological assailants, such as viruses, bacteria, and parasites, which were once the main threats to health; and it is true for what might be termed the "environmental agents"—that is, things either human-made or whose presence has become dangerous through the ways humans use them—which, in the industrial world, are the ascendant threats to health. In relation to the now ubiquitous food chemicals and exhaust fumes and water pollutants and radiation sources, children stand as the red warning flag of the future. The known peril: about double the intake of lead which can leave young children permanently brain-damaged rarely elicits even a passing headache from an adult. The potential peril: Fetal rats are some fifty times more likely than their mothers to succumb to the same dose of certain cancer-causing chemicals.

We are used to diseases that cause coughs, fevers, flushes, spots, and give other immediate cues to their presence. The environmental diseases are not so courteous. "It is simply impossible," Rachel Carson pointed out more than a decade ago, "to predict the effects of lifetime exposure to chemical and physical agents which are not part of the biological experience of man." The environmental diseases, of which cancer is the great example, can lie latent for years until it is too late to control or treat them. Knowing their ends may be largely futile; uncovering their beginnings is the great health challenge of industrial civilization.

The signals children are currently sending back from their precarious vantage point indicate that the environmental toll on well-being is greater both in scope and impact than has been generally understood. Looking for these signals, however, requires a different eye and focus than does looking for the signals of biological disease. Rather than looking for increased childhood deaths, for example, it may be more useful to know whether more children are becoming chronically ill, or whether the age of onset of certain diseases has become lower. Are there new diseases or syndromes? Have the rates of serious or subtle malformations to the fetus changed, and, for that matter, *are* environmental agents proving fatal to these most vulnerable of beings? Pinpointing the beginnings of environmental disease requires going virtually to the beginning of life itself.

✳

Spontaneous miscarriage of an embryo or fetus is not an event that greatly concerns most people. Even a woman who spontaneously loses a wanted child before birth tends to accept this as a mischance of fate. But to geneticists and other biologists, miscarriage is an event of high import. The reason for this is quite simple. Spontaneous abortion occurs through three basic mechanisms— the sperm, the egg, or both forming the conceptus sustained lethal genetic damage; the fetus, after conception, was assaulted by a toxin; or the mother is just not able to carry a child to term. Of these, genetic damage is easily the leading cause of abortion; perhaps one half of spontaneously aborted conceptuses display gross chromosomal damage of a sort geneticists can now "read" under a microscope, and it is presumed another large portion have genetic damage of types not yet decipherable.

By marking an early end to beings who cannot survive in the present world, spontaneous abortion represents a fairly benign form of "natural selection." It is also a rather extraordinary biological fail-safe system, which permits nature to experiment with new genetic traits without having to pay the full price of a live but badly injured human being for any errors made. Any increase above the "natural" rate of miscarriage, however, would be an environmental alarm suggesting that toxic substances were either killing large numbers of fetuses outright or causing new, lethal mutations to their parents' sperm or eggs. Such an artificial increase would not just represent a form of "benign selection"; it would also pose a warning for the living. Many if not most agents that cause abortion early in pregnancy could be expected to leave some surviving babies with injuries; and any mutagens introduced in the world would probably not be so considerate as to lethally jumble a few parents' genes while leaving everyone else's unscathed. In the fly, for example, whose short life cycle and vast numbers of progeny have made it a favored subject for genetic research, the overall "mutation rate is at least fifteen times the lethal mutation rate." In other words, for every impairment to the genes that causes an offspring to die, there are fifteen "minor" gene changes compatible with survival.

The exact number of spontaneous abortions in a population is rather hard to compute for the simple reason that many doomed conceptuses do not survive the few weeks until a woman is aware of a pregnancy. Studying the conceptuses found in the uteri of hysterectomized women has suggested that as many as 30 percent of fertilized eggs may now be in such bad condition that they would easily abort within two weeks.

Yet, even dealing in rough estimates, many people are disconcerted by the amount of fetal loss that is apparently common in the United States. A few years ago, for example, Harold L. Gordon, then medical director of the Dow Chemical Corporation, conceded that, at present, "about 30 to 40 percent of all conceptions usually end in spontaneous abortion, stillbirth, or live birth with congenital malformation, [and] an undetermined number of these are probably the result of some environmental factor."

A few years later, in August 1978, Dr. Gordon's statement received dramatic emphasis. Eight women from small Oregon towns, who had not accepted their miscarriages as mischance, reported to the Environmental Protection Agency that they actually lost their babies soon after local lumber companies, the Federal Bureau of Land Management, and the United States Forest Service had sprayed forests near their homes with a defoliant containing 2,4,5-T. (This substance, of which Dow Chemical is the largest American manufacturer, first attracted controversy when the United States government used it during the war in Vietnam to defoliate thousands of acres of Asian jungle and countryside.) "We are not," wrote Bonnie Hill, a schoolteacher and one of these eight women, "trying to make rash, unsubstantiated claims. But we are interested in seeing if there is a cause-effect relationship. Some of us do know that acreages near our homes and in our water drainages were sprayed within a month before our miscarriages."

In the spring of 1979, the EPA basically concurred with the claim that 2,4,5-T had caused some miscarriages and invoked a temporary emergency ban on some types of 2,4,5-T spraying. Whether this ban will remain in effect against legal challenges from Dow remains to be seen. In the interim, however, it hardly speaks well for the general state of environmental perception that 2,4,5-T was for years annually sprayed on some five million acres—somewhat less than the combined areas of Connecticut, Delware, and Rhode Island—before it was offficially linked to miscarriage. (The Vietnamese had actually complained during the war that some American defoliants were causing both miscarriages and birth defects, but the United States government always denied the charge.) Obviously, 2,4,5-T is but one possible abortifacient (abortion-causing agent) in a world brimming with toxic materials. It is not surprising under these circumstances that, leaving aside stillbirths and malformations, some geneticists now think that "a figure of about 45 percent for the incidence of spontaneous loss" alone is probable.

How such approximate figures for spontaneous abortion compare with the miscarriage rate in former centuries will simply never be known for certain. Assuming, however, that such estimates of the rate of spontaneous loss are fairly correct, adding them to the epidemic death rates from disease that were once the human lot simply does not allow much leeway for people to have produced a replacement population each generation. For this and for other reasons, some geneticists also find it "hard to believe that the human race has successfully endured such [miscarriage] rates over its eight hundred generations."

In concert with the increased awareness of the potential of environmental agents to cause miscarriages, there has also been a dramatic new understanding of the many long-term effects that toxins may inflict on fetuses that do survive. Traditionally, in speaking of "birth defects," both physicians and the general public have meant large and obvious malformations—the missing limbs, clubfeet, cleft palates, fatally jumbled hearts, and improperly closed skulls that are almost immediately apparent in newborns. Probably half or more of these (although the exact proportion is utterly unknown) are the products of spontaneous mutation and cannot be avoided. Another portion may reflect new mutations induced by environmental agents, and still another portion is evidently the work of environmental teratogens, or birth-defect–causing agents, which assault the fetus after conception. (The word *teratogen* comes from the Greek *tera,* meaning "monster." The first syllable is pronounced to rhyme with "rare.") The thalidomide disaster of the late 1950s is probably the most publicized example of an environmental teratogen at work: After their mothers had taken a common tranquilizing agent, several thousand children, most of them European, were left severely disfigured, their limbs partially or entirely missing. In recent years, however, biologists have begun to perceive that environmental agents may leave a fetus with internal damage that, while not obvious in the newborn, may ultimately prove as crucial as even a missing limb, gashed palate, or clubfoot.

A stunning recent realization is that cancer can be induced in the womb. Barely a decade ago, it was not thought that chemicals that had traveled the long, buffering route from the mother's stomach through the placenta could survive in sufficiently concentrated toxicity to produce cancer in the fetus. This belief has since been shattered in the laboratory by the discovery of about a half-hundred chemicals that are transplacental carcinogens (cancer-causing agents that cross the placenta) in unborn animals. And, in 1971, the diagnosis of genital cancers in several young women whose mothers had been prescribed the synthetic hormone DES during their pregnancies first confirmed that transplacental carcinogenesis was a human prospect. These cancers had not appeared soon after birth or even in the childhood years. The first patients were between the ages of fourteen and twenty-two when symptoms of their prenatally induced tumors were finally noticed.

That a baby could leave the womb predisposed toward cancers that may take fifteen, twenty, or more years to surface casts a long perspective over any effort to gauge the environmental damage done in childhood. In the 1950s, cancer, which is often said to be 60 percent or more environmental in origin, became the largest disease killer of children under fifteen in most of the "advanced" world. In the phrase of the late pathologist Paul Michael, this statistic was "both real and relative. Real in the sense that malignant disease has increased both in number and percentage, and relative in that many of the [other] childhood diseases have been controlled successfully by antibiotics, immunizations, and other modern therapies."

The ascendancy of childhood cancer was duly noted but not considered alarming, because the deaths hardly approached the deaths for childhood diseases of previous decades. In 1920, for example, 16,000 American children under age fifteen had died of influenza. Another 12,000 died of tuberculosis. By comparison, the 3,600 cancer deaths that occurred in this same age group a half century later in 1970 do not stand out as crisis figures. But DES and other agents now suspected of transplacental and childhood induction warn that cancer cases in childhood represent only a portion of cancers initiated in early life.

Perhaps more than any similar discovery, transplacental carcinogenesis has caused a profound reassessment of the ways environmental agents may harm a fetus. In the wake of thalidomide, many nations, including the United States, started birth-defect registries, which cover all births or selected sampling areas. It was hoped that registries would pick up trends toward increased malformation before any new teratogens among the some 4 million new substances synthesized each year left behind thousands of victimized children as thalidomide had done.

But registries of severe defects may be misleading as a teratogenic alarm. There are about 2 billion known synthetic and natural chemicals, and clearly, if very many of them caused physical or "structural" abnormalities, few normal-looking babies would ever be born. But severe birth defects are a relatively infrequent occurrence. Most nations report a birth defect rate ranging between 3 and 6 percent of live births, depending somewhat on the completeness of their statistics and the defects they count as "severe." By contrast, both laboratory and clinical work indicate that there is little boundary to the chemical potential to leave the fetus with slight yet crucial "substructural" flaws, which may later show themselves as "functional" defects—say, as general ill health, or as the failure of such biochemical arrangements as the immune and enzyme systems. Over and over again, however, the message from experimental work with chemical after chemical is that the brain is predominantly the first place to falter "slightly" in the face of a "slight" environmental assault on the fetus.

Methylmercury is a toxic compound that has already achieved notoriety as the cause of Minamata disease, a crippling and sometimes fatal degeneration of the central nervous system, first noticed among Japanese who had eaten fish contaminated with mercury wastes discharged into Minamata Bay by a local industry. Many people are familiar with the late Eugene Smith's haunting photographs of children who were severely deformed when their mothers ate contaminated fish during pregnancy. Fewer people are aware that, in some areas of Minamata, upward of 25 percent of local school children—about double to triple the usual rates in Japan—are considered "mentally deficient" even though they are quite normal in their outward appearance. There is some question whether their injury will end with varying degrees of mental deficiency or whether worse awaits some, or all, of these children. Experimental work has strongly suggested that even relatively slight early brain damage from methylmercury becomes more and more distressful as times goes by.

Joan Spyker, now director of Interdisciplinary Toxicology at the University of Arkansas Medical School, is a woman with waist-length brown hair and a profound interest in the causation of mental and nervous distress. After beginning her working life as a physical therapist for brain-damaged children, she became more and more preoccupied with "finding out what had really happened to those kids," and returned to medical school. In the early 1970s, Dr. Spyker and methylmercury came together in a series of experiments that strikingly detail the range of functions at stake in prenatal encounters.

Joan Spyker injected pregnant mice with a dose of mercury well below that needed to provoke physical abnormality—actually an innocuous dose by the toxicological standards of even a few years ago. From their birth until about a year and a half later, a time passage marking a comfortable middle age in the mouse life cycle, the young mercury-exposed mice did not outwardly appear to be different from unexposed control mice raised beside them. Testing, however, brought out a health problem. Many of the mercury mice had contracted severe infections, including pneumonia. To Dr. Spyker, this finding was "entirely unexpected" and pointed to the conclusion that "impaired immune function may indeed be a delayed effect of prenatal exposure to methylmercury."

On the way past middle age, the mercury mice lost even their outward claim to normalcy. Their muscles atrophied and, postures sagging, they fast deteriorated into a catalogue of geriatric complaints. Some went blind and a few abruptly doubled in weight. As it is well known that mercury concentrates in the fetal brain, it was assumed their sorry condition somehow related to brain damage they had sustained prenatally, but examination of these mouse brains under an ordinary light microscope did not reveal any structural harm. Only when the brains were subjected to the inquisition of an electron microscope, at which point they were magnified 48,000 times, was damage revealed—damage so slight it was virtually confined to individual cells. Yet these small flaws seem to have been sufficient to disqualify the test animals from gracefully withstanding a lifetime of activity, stress, and mousely concerns. (In the constant illustration of the desperate susceptibility of the fetus, the maternal mice, who had encountered the very same dose of mercury, just lived out their lives in an ordinary fashion, unbothered by sagging muscles, blindness, and sudden obesity.)

Dosages are not really comparable between mice and humans, but certainly the symptoms in Minamata victims have been similar, with many of the exposed Japanese villagers displaying vision and hearing losses, tremors, and incoordination—and some dying prematurely. Scientists ordinarily decline to assign specifically human traits to animal results, but in the instance at hand, Dr. Spyker says she has "no hesitation about calling these animals senile because there actually is a direct human model. As they get older, victims of Minamata are deteriorating in just the ways the animal model predicted they would."

Of course, it is hardly as simple to monitor the toxic

exposures of human children as it is to monitor those of laboratory mice administered a carefully measured excess of a single toxin. Nonetheless, through all the variety of human toxic exposures, epidemiological probing (epidemiology is the study of disease patterns and causation in populations) has now managed to suggest that prenatal exposures to appropriate chemicals may sometimes permanently alter even those mystical traits that render humans peculiarly human—traits such as "behavior," "conduct," and the vagaries of personal feeling. In 1977, for example, researchers at the University of British Columbia asked the teachers of more than 300 six-and-a-half-year-olds to rate the kids' behavior. The teachers—who, by the way, were unaware of the purpose of the rating—considered children whose mothers had smoked during the pregnancy to be a little more troublesome than children whose mothers had not smoked. In the cautious way that scientific researchers tend to express themselves, it was decided that "some slight damaging effect of maternal smoking during pregnancy on the fetal brain development and subsequent behavior . . . cannot be excluded."

Moving from outward perceptions of behavior to the internal graces of feeling, attitude, and sentiment, Dr. June Reinisch, a behavioral endocrinologist at Rutgers University, thought to administer standard personality tests to children whose mothers had been prescribed sex hormones, in the form of synthetic estrogens or progestins, during the first six months of pregnancy. From the late 1940s until the early 1970s, these substances were widely administered as "hormone supports" to pregnancy. It was believed that they guarded against miscarriage, premature onset of labor, poor fetal growth, and other lapses. Rather late in the day, epidemiological follow-up not only failed to document any improvement in pregnancy outcome among women who had used hormones, but uncovered numbers of physical problems among children who had been exposed to them. DES, the most popular of the various estrogen preparations, turned out to be a transplacental carcinogen. And both estrogens and progestins have been implicated to some extent in causing heart defects, "limb reduction" deformities (full or partial loss of the limbs or extremities), and various confusions of sexual development.

It is more obvious today why Dr. Reinisch started looking for personality changes in the exposed children than it was at the time. By the late 1950s, it was well known that some girls exposed to progestins were being born with "ambiguous genitalia" or even a rudimentary penis. The romance with pregnancy supports was so intense at that point, however, that a matter of a penis on the wrong sex hardly caused the appropriate second thoughts. The defect was relatively infrequent and seemed to be limited to a few products, which were withdrawn from the market. There was a general assumption that since these little girls otherwise appeared to be normal and to possess their female reproductive organs, they would grow up, have sex, and have children. The medical literature of the time described their "pseudohermaphroditism" as being "easily corrected" by "simple amputation of the phallus" and, sometimes, a little "reconstructive surgery." The standard advice of the day was just to carefully check progestin-exposed children lest girls raised as boys startle everyone when they began to menstruate in adolescence.

Probably most of these girls did mature to have reasonably normal lives. What went unmentioned, however, is that one thing lost by growing a penis is the clitoris—the female phallus. This loss in itself does not forbid sex or even sensual pleasure—just full sexual response; but for some of these young women, intercourse will always be painful because of the scar tissue left by their simple "reconstructive surgery."

In the past few years, surveys of grown DES sons have confirmed that about one quarter of them also sustained genital abnormalities, including, in some cases, microphallus (a condition defined as a penis of less than 1½ inches—4 centimeters—when not erect). It is probably unfortunate that the genital abnormalities of boy babies were not the first problems with pregnancy supports to claim attention. If the mostly male medical world of the 1950s seems to have had some rather blithe ideas about how easy it would be to "correct" the female genital tract, no one would have made the same assumption about microphallus, a condition that is simply not correctable. Confronted with this conclusive damage, doctors might well have grown wary about pregnancy supports much sooner.

Part of the reason for these abnormalities is that the sex hormones, although thought of as being "male" or "female," are remarkably similar in chemical structure. Progesterone, the natural hormone progestins were intended to mimic, is known as "the hormone of pregnancy." It maintains pregnancy and stimulates lactation; but it is also the chemical precursor of the androgens, the male sex hormones. Meanwhile, the androgens and the estrogens, the female sex hormones, are so closely related that both sexes of many mammal species can convert one to the other inside their bodies.

The mistake made in synthetically mimicking progesterone was that some of the products were a little too "androgenic." Dr. Reinisch wondered whether there had been a more general but subtle impact on the central nervous system even when children escaped obvious abnormality. In useful if chauvinistic terms, the heightened androgenic character of the synthetic progestins could be expected to bring out aggression and self-assertion in children, while estrogen could be expected to bring out their quietness, shyness, and "femininity." Only one of the seventy-one children Reinisch tested was visibly malformed—a little girl missing fingers and toes. But when she compared the personality tests of both the estrogen-exposed children and progestin-exposed children with one another—and with their own brothers and sisters—they fell into distinct categories. The progestin-exposed boys and girls revealed themselves to be "more independent and individualistic, more self-assured and self-sufficient" than the estrogen children and their own siblings. By contrast, the estrogen-exposed children were more group-oriented and less independent. This does not, in any sense, imply that these children are headed for the psychiatrist's couch or mental institutions. What it does mean is that within a fairly normal personality range, they turned up closer to one end of the scale than is usual. "It is not unexpected," Dr.

Reinisch has commented, "that a difference in personality would exist between hormone-exposed and unexposed siblings as well as between treatments. The animal research of the past decade and a half indicates that early exposure to hormones . . . affects a wide range of behaviors including activity level, social interaction, curiosity, emotionality, dominance, and aggression."

In the twenty-five years of their use, synthetic estrogens were prescribed to between 250,000 and 3 million pregnant women— the latter figure being the Department of Health, Education and Welfare's most recent "outside projection." In 1971, when the carcinogenicity of DES was discovered, there was a great switch to progestins. Over the next three years, until the Food and Drug Administration withdrew approval of all hormone supports during pregnancy, about 500,000 prescriptions were written annually for progestin use during pregnancy. Already the consequences to children have ranged from cancer to, perhaps, subtle alterations of personality. It will be an intriguing, if morbid, lesson in environmental insight to learn what else these children reveal about themselves as the years go by—these children, slapped on the buttocks and pronounced perfectly fine at birth.

As prenatal life is left behind, this desperate vulnerability is also left. But young and growing bodies do generally remain more susceptible to environmental agents than do adult bodies. The characteristic effects of air pollution are a case in point. In much of the advanced world, respiratory disease, which is closely linked with some air pollutants, now takes second place only to cancer as a disease killer of children under age fifteen. Air-pollution episodes are especially dangerous for infants. Their lungs must struggle against befouled air with an aerating surface relative to body weight smaller than that of both older children and adults. In the Great London Smog of 1952, the death rate for children under one year of age doubled. An analysis of 1970 infant mortality in Dauphin County, Pennsylvania, similarly pinpointed the deaths of

26 of the 66 babies born that year who did not reach their first birthday to a thirty-one-day period when the county was shrouded in intense air pollution or, as the *New York Times* put it, in a "hot, muggy blanket of smoggy air."

Again, however, trying to gauge the toll of environmental agents by counting immediate deaths can be misleading. The long-term impact of air pollution on the young is evidently severe enough that even an adulthood spent in clean air does not fully rescind a childhood spent in dirty air. The New Zealand National Health Service, for one, has reported that immigrants from England, the country abjured in poem for its "dark, satanic mills," have a 30 percent higher death rate from lung cancer than do native whites; and when immigrants leave England after age thirty, their chance of dying from lung cancer vaults even higher, to 75 percent more than that of native whites.

Respiratory illness also seems to have become the major chronic disease of industrialized childhood; in the United States, it now accounts for about 60 percent of total school days lost to illness and, in the particular form of asthma, has sentenced more and more of the young to the sad world of constant illness. An association with pollen once gave asthma the popular, if not fully accurate, reputation of being a country hazard, but its growth in urban areas has been staggering. As the Chairman of the Department of Pediatrics at Montefiore Hospital, a facility in the Bronx that is part of New York City's second-largest medical complex, Dr. Laurence Finberg has been a close observer of urban health patterns. "Those of us who trained in pediatrics two or three decades ago," he told a 1975 conference on pediatrics and the environment, "did not in our training years think of the management of asthmatic children as occupying a major portion of our emergency room experience. Today, in a large city's hospital emergency rooms, such care leads over almost all other diagnostic categories."

Before New York began to enforce new laws controlling incinerators and the sulphur content of fuel coal, the asthma epidemic had attained such severity that some children died of the disease. The fatalities tapered off around 1975, but there is still concern about the virulence of contemporary asthma attacks. "It's something that's hard to document," Dr. Finberg comments on his "feeling" that asthma cases today are often more severe than they once were, "but you just get a sense of these things from your clinical experience. In any case, I certainly do not remember thinking of asthma as a potentially fatal condition when I was a resident, and yet we had started to lose a few children to it each year."

In a typical recent emergency case at North Bronx Medical Center, an affiliate of Montefiore, a little boy named Duvaughn who was just two months short of his third birthday was brought in by his mother. It was his second hospital admission for asthma in his young life, and his 31 pounds seemed to embody all the medical and social stress that asthma now claims. Duvaughn was almost prostrate from the effort to breathe. Toward the end of an asthma attack, the airways narrow, making it harder to breathe out than to breathe in. The chest enlarges, and, comments Dr. Richard Kravath, a lung specialist at Montefiore, the child "has to work really hard." Duvaughn's little stomach, pumping up and down in desperation, looked rather like a balloon riding a seesaw. After several hours in the emergency room, where preliminary measures to halt the attack had not worked, Duvaughn was admitted to North Bronx and tucked in a crib, an intravenous needle in his arm, his soft brown eyes glazed over, and his mother standing by. "I'm always afraid I'm going to lose him," she said.

It is often no easier to unravel the causes of an emphatic disease like asthma, which propels many young patients to emergency rooms, than to unravel the causes of cancers that have been latent for twenty or thirty years. About 200 million tons of toxic materials, 60 percent of them from the engines of motor vehicles, are released into the atmosphere of the United States every year. While some of these materials—notably the amount of sulphate in fuel oil and fuel coal—seem more crucial than others to the onset of asthma attacks, equations between precise pollutants and asthma will probably remain obscure. There are also, of course, numerous causes of asthma besides pollutants. Psychological stress, the common cold, allergy, and even nuances of lifestyle may leave some children under attack and struggling for breath.

Even a few childhood cases of an illness once considered to represent decades of wear and tear and to be the sole property of adults may be an alarm signal for environmental disease. The children either most genetically sensitive or most proximately exposed to a toxin may be the first to become ill, but their sickness holds a threat that other cases may follow. It may or may not be important, for example, that the Hamman-Rich syndrome, an often fatal form of pulmonary fibrosis (scarring of the lung tissue), which used to be almost unheard of among children, is now claiming an occasional child victim. In two childhood cases seen at Montefiore in recent years, the children—one lived and one died—had experienced a recent encounter with paraquat, an herbicide that came on the market in the mid-1960s. Two cases, of course, do not make for a conclusion or even for a trend; but they are something to be aware of should there be a large increase in the incidence of childhood Hamman-Rich syndrome.

On the other hand, it is unquestionably important that the age of onset for heart disease in the United States and much of the Western world has now lowered to the point that no one raises an eyebrow to hear about heart attack victims in their thirties or forties. The epidemic incidence of heart disease has largely been blamed on sedentary habits, fatty diet, and cigarette smoking. But in 1973, Dr. Milton Zaret, a Scarsdale, New York, ophthalmologist, proposed that another factor might be a part of the heart-disease equation. The number of microwave-induced cataracts that Dr. Zaret was seeing in his eye practice prompted him some years ago to research extensively the side effects of microwave radiation. He has proposed that in much the same way that microwave damage to the elasticity of the lens capsule could explain these cataracts, microwave strain on the internal elastic membrane of the cardiovascular system could contribute to heart failure. In view of the myriad uses of microwaves in industrial societies, this is no small proposal. Sweeping continuously from radar installations, bouncing international Olympic coverage from space satellites, sending television signals, and cooking food, microwaves at various levels have become an intimate, not to say unavoidable, companion to everyday life.

Zaret's theory was not based on his practice alone. His interest in microwaves had alerted him to the plight of North Karelia and Kuopio, two rural districts of Finland, which, throughout most of the 1970s—and to the bafflement of the medical community—have sustained the highest rate of heart attack in the world. They are not polluted areas; their populations are largely engaged in lumbering, farming, and other nonsedentary work; and their vast, silent forests would seem to hold out a promise of wholesome serenity.

North Karelia and Kuopio are, however, across a large lake from the Soviet Union—and from a major Soviet radar installation. (Radar aims microwaves at targets in short bursts.) This unit is aimed at the American Midwest and is intended to detect missiles launched from underground silos there, but the immediate "enhancing" effect of the lake on the microwaves would presumably put North Karelia and Kuopio into unusual jeopardy. The heart attack rate in these two districts rises the closer the individual homes are to the Soviet border and, in North Karelia and Kuopio, fatal heart attacks are not uncommon among men in their twenties. Zaret's theory is controversial; but whether or not it turns out to be correct, it does emphasize that situations that involve unusual age distributions of disease demand to be looked at in unusual ways. It is hard to explain these young heart attack victims with the conventional accusations against cigarette smoking and butter consumption.

Biology does not always send so obvious a message as a heart attack. A trend now also commanding attention concerns children whose problems may seem trivial by comparison to malformations, heart attacks, genital cancers, and even asthma. These are children who are just unusually nervous or overexcitable. They are grouped under such vague labels as "hyperactive" or "minimally brain damaged" or "learning disabled"—little-understood problems that concern behavior, coordination, and other functional abilities. Hyperactive children may have a genius IQ but not be able to concentrate long enough to learn to read; they may otherwise appear quite healthy, but not possess the motor control to grasp a pencil firmly. Semi-official and official sources now estimate that as many as one, two, or even five million American children are subject to such conditions—although these numbers are among the more hotly disputed health statistics. The trouble in estimating the incidence of "functional" defects is that their diagnosis is largely based on opinion and observation rather than measurable signs such as degrees of fever, heartbeats per minute, or blood counts. A child one pediatrician calls "hyperactive" may stand before the next pediatrician as a mere brat.

Some children are just born that way, and others are made that way by various causes, among them psychological trauma, outright abuse, brain damage at birth, hypoglycemia, and severe allergies to natural foods. Increasingly, however, reports in the medical and scientific literature have suggested that environmental agents are deeply implicated in the causation of such syndromes. In human children—in addition to prenatal exposure to cigarettes—lead, copper, synthetic food additives, trace metals, and certain types of fluorescent lighting have all been cited as causing or contributing to behavior and learning effects. Young monkeys nursed by mothers who had been given PCBs in their food are also hyperactive in behavior. Now restricted, PCBs (polychlorinated biphenyls) were formerly used as everything from a pesticide extender to a component of "carbonless" carbon paper, and are still a persistent environmental contaminant; in the monkey experiments the PCB level was only notches above that routinely measured in human breast milk.

This steady identification of a variety of chemicals as contributors to "minimal brain damage," odd behavior, and learning deficits promises to stand as a real turning point in the comprehension of environmental disease. These children may well represent a kind of "pre-warning system" about environmental contamination. Over and over again in the laboratory, it has turned out that slight quirks of behavior, learning, and conduct in the young animal are the first signs of latent nervous-system damage that will later cause serious deterioration in the adult animal—deterioration, for example, along the lines of that seen in Spyker's mercury-exposed mice. And both the mass of children said to be affected and the variety of agents involved suggest something very crucial about the regulation of toxins—that the traditional method of setting individual safety standards for single pesticides, separate chemicals, and lone additives is wrong. These children suggest that the combined impact of environmental chemicals eminently requires attention. Pollution, of course, is a worldwide problem, but it has mighty excesses in the United States. In a country where each person annually consumes some two pounds of synthetic food chemicals; where the level of BHT, a common preservative, measured in human fatty tissues is six times that measured in British citizens; where some 6 percent of the children tested each year have "undue" lead absorption; and where the concentration of radio waves over some urban areas is 100 to 200 million times what the sun itself emanates, the immature nervous systems of the young are at risk of simply being overwhelmed by the pollutants around them.

It so often turns out that common chemical exposures that may mean nothing to adults are injurious to children, that some people think we must reform our whole attitude toward toxins and regulation. A person who thinks so emphatically is Dr. Robert Miller, offficially chief of the Clinical Epidemiology Branch of the National Cancer Institute, but personally more interested in the full spectrum of environmental disease. From 1973 to 1979, he headed the Environmental Hazards Committee of The American Academy of Pediatrics. A soft-spoken, precise man with a preference for bow ties, Dr. Miller began his medical life as a pediatrician. He recalls his interest in children and the environment beginning when, as a resident, he became aware of the radiation doses being sustained by infants. In those days, it was common for doctors to fluoroscope infants and children rather than X ray them. The fluoroscope, which is something of radiology's equivalent of a moving picture camera, allowed doctors to take a constant look at fidgety children rather than trying to make them sit still for X-ray pictures. The doses, however, were much higher than those of ordinary X rays. (Many people may remember when a trip to the shoe store included the chance to watch your toes wiggle under a fluoroscope.)

Dr. Miller's idea is that there should be a special government agency that does nothing but try to limit unnecessary childhood exposure to toxins. "Take something like fireproofed mattresses," he says. "Of course, they're intended to keep adults who smoke from burning themselves up in bed, but what about premature babies in incubators? They sweat and urinate and are more or less soaking up a chemical that's not protecting them from anything. We should just look at everything twice to see possible effects on children."

In rough outline, then, these are some of the manifestations of environmental disease among the young that have been, to some extent, noticed and documented. It is obvious that environmental disease represents a challenge quite different from that of biological diseases of childhood. Environmental diseases are more insidious. As seen with DES cancers and the mercury-exposed mice, they tend to inflict long-term damage without even having the courtesy to announce clear symptoms in the present. They tend to damage children at levels of toxic exposure far below the levels needed to cause similar damage to adults. Environmental diseases do not characteristically yield to "total" recoveries even when treated. There is no way, for example, to put back fingers and toes that never grew in the womb or to replace injured brain cells or to "cure" asthma.

There could hardly be a greater health mission than to fill in this outline with specific counts of disease and precise agents at fault; there could also hardly be a more complex one. Once the laboratory is left behind for the muddled, whirling world of human subjects, causation, incidence, accurate diagnosis, chemical intake, and exposure become almost hopelessly intertwined. If chemicals not infrequently conduct themselves like hyperactive seven-year-olds, taking abrupt turns and twists that no one foresaw from their chemical formulations or their laboratory behavior, statistics are often confusing or deceiving. Perhaps no incident better illustrates the problem of trying to gather what would seem to be the most basic, simple information than the recent controversy over Down's syndrome and maternal age.

Down's syndrome is a birth defect whose incidence medicine watches very closely. Once known as "mongolism" for the broad, flat facial features common to its victims, Down's syndrome invariably signals the loss of normal intelligence. The standard mechanism for its occurrence is that the child has three twenty-first chromosomes instead of the normal two. Usually when genetic damage is so great that the chromosomes break, or divide wrongly, or are otherwise in major error, the conceptus aborts. Although easily the majority of Down's conceptions end in miscarriage, more Down's fetuses do survive to be born than is customary after chromosome damage. About fourteen out of every ten thousand live-born infants in the general population have Down's syndrome.

Its role as a genetic harbinger would be enough in itself to assure a fascination with Down's syndrome, but, additionally, Down's syndrome has the fairly unusual habit of increasing in incidence with the age of the mother. A teratological rule of thumb, stated in text after text, is that mothers "over age thirty-five constitute only 13.5 percent of all pregnancies, but they produce over 50 percent of all infants with mongolism." This age progression may well represent a specific process of deterioration in the maternal egg—a process that environmental agents, conceivably, could hasten. An often overlooked feature of the female mammal is that, for reproductive purposes at least, her body arrives in the world complete, a lifetime supply of eggs already present. The human female's ovaries contain at birth some two million oocytes (immature eggs), of which 400 are eventually released during the reproductive years. An average man can produce about 100 million new sperm cells every day; but, for the woman, these two million reproductive or "germ" cells are a lifetime's quota. Losses are not replaced.

A woman's oocytes-in-waiting are in the uncomfortable position of being virtually lifetime targets for environmental toxins. There have been repeated research efforts in the United States and elsewhere to identify agents that could specifically provoke Down's syndrome; but, with the exception of several studies that found that the chances for the disorder rise somewhat with the number of abdominal X rays a woman has before conception, little has been discovered about the possible role of the outside environment in causing this syndrome. In fact, simple counts of the numbers of Down's infants have shown nothing alarming. In country after country, both defect registries and specific studies have found recent rates of Down's births to be steady, or even to have slightly declined. In the Canadian province of British Columbia, for one place, between 1952 and 1973, Down's incidence declined from 1.384 to 1.146 per 1,000 live births and, among those hospitals in the western United States that report to the Birth Defects Monitoring Program of the federal Public Health Service, the drop between 1970 and 1975 was from 1.25 to 0.75 per 1,000 total births.

On the surface, then, it seemed that even a world synthesizing four million new chemicals a year, swallowing drugs by the gross, and spreading microwaves by untold intensities was still pretty safe from severe chromosome damage—or, at least, chromosome damage compatible with live births. But in 1970 Irene Uchida, a Canadian epidemiologist who had been studying Down's births in the province of Manitoba, reported that the mean age of the mothers of these children had dropped by five years between 1960 and 1967; by 1967 their mean age was twenty-nine. This age plunge, Uchida proposed, might "indicate that important environmental factors" had begun to operate in the causation of Down's syndrome. Similar reports of a drop in the age at which women are conceiving Down's children have since come from Sweden, Japan, New Zealand, and the Canadian province of British Columbia. The Department of Epidemiology of the New York State Department of Health, an unusually imaginative outpost of state bureaucracy, in what seems to be the only American figures on this question has reported "a noticeable and consistent shift downward in maternal age" of New York State Down's mothers. Only from Australia has there been a survey that did not note a significant decline in the age of Down's mothers. But the Australian survey is somewhat earlier than the rest, covering the relatively chemical-free years of 1942 to 1957.*

Why, then, didn't the increased number of Down's babies being born to young women show up as an increase in the overall rate of Down's babies? A closer look at the British Columbia figures suggests how even the most straightforward sorts of statistics deceive. What had also changed during the time of these surveys was the willingness of older women to have any children at all. Freed by reliable contraceptives, they removed themselves from motherhood by the millions and, during the twenty-one year period studied, the mean maternal age of *all* mothers in British Columbia declined by two and one half years. Had this shrinkage in the population "naturally" expected to conceive the most Down's babies perhaps balanced out an increase in environmentally related cases? In the estimate of a University of British Columbia research team, a 23 percent decrease in Down's children should have accompanied this change in mean maternal age—not the paltry 4 percent decrease that actually occurred. Meanwhile, the mean age at which women were conceiving Down's children was dropping *three times* as fast as the overall maternal age. The births to younger women were replacing those "lost" as older women stopped having children and, possibly, a statistical limbo had disguised an important environmentally rooted *increase* in Down's babies.

Some commentators are not convinced of the environmental explanation for these numbers. They think the explanation may lie

---

* In recent years, it has been widely recommended that older mothers have amniocentesis, a method of prenatal diagnosis to determine whether they are carrying a Down's fetus. If they are, many choose to abort. This has further lowered the age of Down's mothers, but it does not account for the age changes in these reports, which were all made before amniocentesis became generally available.

in the improved diagnosis of Down's syndrome in recent years—especially techniques of chromosome analysis, which spot Down's children whose facial and physical features do not immediately give them away. To other observers, the change in the age of Down's mothers, from the pristine stretches of British Columbia to the polluted confines of Japan, represents a stern warning that industrial society may have set loose any number of agents—pesticides, radio waves, oral contraceptives—whose biological toll it has profoundly failed to understand. Or, as the Swedes judiciously put the matter, "a combination of the two explanations may, of course, also exist." What is clear for the moment is that the most closely watched statistics cannot be depended upon to catch even large changes of course.

Down's syndrome, like other forms of genetic damage, relates to perhaps the most crucial question of all—the specter of an increased rate of genetic mutation. Cancer, brain damage, and birth defects caused by direct-acting agents do, after all, finally die with the life they have plagued. Mutation threatens not only children now being conceived, but the destiny of the species; it threatens, in the phrase of one scientist, "the *sine qua non* of all that we value and all that we are."

Geneticists generally believe that any artificial increase in the rate of mutation is undesirable. This is because most mutations are to some degree harmful; they can be expected to provoke anything from fatal genetic diseases and malformations (sickle-cell anemia, hemophilia, and achondroplastic dwarfism are a few among hundreds of examples) to slight losses in intelligence or disease resistance or just zest for living.

Ironically, substances that are mildly mutagenic are more dangerous than those that announce themselves in lethal or disfiguring disease. "Mild" mutagens are particularly hard to detect and particularly likely to be passed down the generations. The prominent geneticist James Crow, Professor of Medical Genetics at the University of Wisconsin at Madison, has emphasized their potential for "the slow contamination of the gene pool." Especially threatening, a *Medical World News* summary of his observations points out, "would be the introduction of a mildly mutagenic substance, such as an additive to a food or beverage that is mass-produced for wide consumption . . . such a slight increase in man's quotient of bad seed could not in any way be detected. The first warning of such an event might be an increase in the number, incidence or severity of genetic illnesses; marked changes in the birth ratio of men to women; or an almost imperceptible loss of vigor and vitality progressing from generation to generation."

Is this occurring? While breakthroughs in the ability to mass-monitor mutation rates in living populations are expected almost with the next breath science takes, at present the human mutation rate is a matter of argument. On the one hand, so many substances in widespread use—condensate of cigarette smoke, saccharin, the preservative nitrite, hair-dye ingredients—have tested as mutagens on bacteria, flies, rodents, and other organisms, that it seems folly to hope humans have been entirely spared; of course, to some geneticists the current miscarriage rate is one of the stronger indications that we have not been. The late Nobel laureate and geneticist Herman J. Muller, who, in 1927, made what was then the breakthrough discovery of radiation's mutagenicity, spoke for a considerable amount of scientific thought, and still does, in conjuring a future world whose inhabitants would be "devoted chiefly to the effort to live carefully, to spare and prop up their own feebleness, to soothe their inner disharmonies and, in general, to doctor themselves as effectively as possible. For everyone would be an invalid with his own special familial twists. . . ." On the other hand, recent developments, among them evidence that the repair mechanisms of human genes are superior to those of common test species, have, in the delicate phrase of James V. Neel, Chairman of the Department of Human Genetics at the University of Michigan at Ann Arbor, "made us more cautious in predicting the impact on populations of an increased mutation rate."

These are not, of course, pleasant things to think about, but thinking about them in the context of time takes away some of the sting. Curious as it may seem, complete "perfection" among living progeny is not desirable. At least in regard to those defects and disorders that express new mutations, it seems that nature, in her paradox, requires both success and failure, the admirable and the aberration. Mutations, whether good, bad, or indifferent, occur at random. The environment in which people find themselves enhances the survival of those beings with mutation-induced characteristics suited to it. This process of random mutation and environmental selection accounts for species' becoming adapted to changing environments.

Through this slow, cumulative process, humans may eventually become rather impervious to their chemical surroundings—not unlike certain mutant bacteria, which, instead of being killed by antibiotics, actually require them to live. James Neel has used this apparent impossibility of attaining the good without the bad to argue that there "may be a malformation frequency representing the optimum balance between, on the one hand, fetal loss and physical handicap from congenital defects and, on the other hand, population gain from those very same genes which in certain combinations may result in physical defects." The essayist Joan Didion, writing in another context, put the question more succinctly. "Again," she has observed, "it is a question of recognizing that anything worth having has its price."

The point, then, is not to avoid the fact that having children sometimes ends in failure or involves tragedy; it is merely to ensure that industrial civilization does not, in the present, increase the usual problems or cast a long shadow over future generations. Dealing with this problem remains basically a matter of tried and true and plodding methods. It means a steady commitment to researching toxins, carcinogens, and teratogens. It means an accompanying commitment to legislation or other methods of preventing them from wreaking their particular damage on young bodies. The information now available may not be particularly good or complete, but, piecing together what is available from animal studies and human monitoring, from the little secrets of cells to ghastly blunders of development, it suggests plenty of trouble ahead.

> It appears to me necessary to every physician to be skilled in nature, and to strive to know, if he would wish to perform his duties, what man is in relation to the articles of food and drink, and to his other occupations, and what are the effects of each of them to every one.
>
> HIPPOCRATES

# Chapter 2

# BIRTH DEFECTS: OLD AND NEW

In 1976, when she awoke from the anesthesia after delivering her first child, there was a nurse standing by Elizabeth Fletcher's bed. Naturally Mrs. Fletcher, who is a Brooklyn, New York, housewife, inquired after the baby. She received a three-syllable response. "The nurse said, 'Um, um, um,'" she recalls, "and ran to get the doctor. The doctor came in and said something about 'spina bifida.' Next they brought the baby in with a priest. Then they took him out into the hall, baptized him, and took him away. I was so scared. Naturally, I thought he was going to die."

The baby, Edward Fletcher, had spina bifida, a defect characterized by greater or lesser portions of the spinal column failing to close. It may leave children severely crippled in body and in mind. Spina bifida is one of the defects generally lumped under the term "neural tube defects." As a group, these defects are thought to be set off within the first three or four weeks of pregnancy and to result from aberrations in the formation of the neural tube, the embryonic precursor of the central nervous system. They also include anencephaly, in which the forebrain fails to develop, and hydrocephaly, more commonly known as "water on the brain." Anencephaly invariably results in death within a few hours of the child's delivery; spina bifida and hydrocephaly are often to some degree surgically correctable.

"In very few countries," comments a World Health Organization report, "do the neural tube defects constitute less than 10 percent of all major malformations and they contribute a high proportion of those determining stillbirth and early death—overall, more than 50 percent of such deaths." In the developed countries, however, enough advanced care is now available that, with rehabilitation and often with extensive surgery, the prognosis for these children can be quite acceptable—as, indeed, it now is for some other types of birth defects once considered totally devastating. The Fletchers, like the parents of many such children, were first told their son would be "a vegetable." But Edward now walks with crutches. He goes to school and plays with ordinary children and other crippled children alike. From her experience with spina bifida children, Mrs. Fletcher now thinks that many of them are more alert, not to say brighter, than the average child. "They observe a lot," she comments. "It's a form of compensation."

As great, however, as have been the advances in helping many children with birth defects, it still is not easy. "Medically, socially, and educationally, it's a struggle all the way," comments Debbie Scopelitis, another mother of a spina bifida child. "Too often the parents are struggling by themselves. Even doctors often don't know much about it and they can't tell you where to get supports and services." Louise Nachshen points out that her son, Steven, had at least seven operations by the time he was three. The preference, clearly, lies in learning how to avoid severe pre-birth injuries.

But, in their individual distress, the spina bifida children are emblematic of a huge scientific stalemate. From ancient times to the present, few things have so seriously preoccupied the human mind as determining the cause of malformations. To the ancient Babylonians and Sumerians, malformations represented a prediction of events to come; to Christian civilizations, they have often represented "the anger of God or the active intervention of the devil," and a reason to execute both the offending mother and child. In the early twentieth century, when genetics became the new toy of the rational mind, all malformation was assigned to "faults of heredity." In the early 1940s, a series of experiments by the pioneering American teratologist Josef Warkany, which showed that nutritional deprivation would produce various abnormalities in fetal rodents, focused attention on environmental teratogens. Since then there has been a growing belief among both scientists and the public that research will eventually unravel what portion of birth defects is caused by inevitable mutations and what portion is environmental—and find causes for the latter.

As is perhaps natural because of the sorrow and the horror they invoke, the "major defects"—Down's syndrome, neural tube aberrations, cleft lips and palates, limb reduction deformities, and a half dozen others—have been the central objects of this research effort; they have captured the bulk of money devoted to investigating environmental perils to the fetus; they are the focus of endless laboratory exercises, which see rodent, rabbit, monkey, and guinea pig fetuses subjected to chemical after chemical; and they star in epidemiological surveys. By now, the total worldwide effort to unlock the causes of major malformation probably adds up to some tidy billions of dollars.

It has been a major disappointment. By the early 1970s, whatever else may have been seen in animal experiments, only a few important chemical- or drug-induced teratogenic processes—among them sex hormones and genital defects, and alcoholism and mental retardation—had been confirmed in the human population. More important, scientists had not been able to understand why some agents are teratogenic and why others are not; there had been no substantial insight into the chemical or molecular properties that might render various substances a danger to the unborn. Actually, after thirty years, several billions of dollars, and an intensity of effort perhaps exceeded only by the search for a cancer cure, it was hard to say that the contemporary world had much advanced over the Sumerian soothsayers in its interpretation of birth defects. Speaking for the general bewilderment, the American teratologist James Wilson estimated in 1973 that perhaps 25 percent of developmental defects in humans could be attributed to mutation or chromosome aberrations and that another 5 to 8 percent had known"environmental" causes—including biological agents such as viruses. Dr. Wilson pointed out that many people suspect a large portion of the rest resulted from "complex interactions of genetic predisposition and subtle factors in the environment"; but, suspicions aside, the real cause of 65 to 75 percent of birth defects was still unknown.

Why had it been so frustrating to link malformations to causes? On the surface, there appeared a simple logic in beginning at the beginning. According to epidemiological theory, by either taking populations exposed to a certain agent and watching their future health, or taking a health condition and working backward to find environmental exposures peculiar to its victims, an understanding of causation should advance at a steady clip. In reality, the unknowns and variables of lives lived outside a laboratory stand like a contingent of surly guards, blocking teratological researchers at every turn. There is perhaps no more graphic illustration of how, out in the field, promising situations fade to nothing than the twenty-year saga of neural tube defects and local water supply.

Of the major defects, the neural tube malformations seemed to hold a special promise of yielding, at least partly, to an environmental solution. In animals, any number of factors, among them vitamin and trace-metal overdoses and diet deficiencies, had been shown to drastically impair the neural tube development of the fetus. In humans, the occurrence pattern of neural tube defects suggested it was quite possible they did result from an interaction of "genetic predisposition and subtle factors in the environment." Both Japanese children living in Hawaii and non-Welsh children living in Wales, for example, have a different rate of neural tube malformations than native children; their rate lies between the rate usual for their ethnic group and that of their place of residence. In the United States and in Canada, rates along the East Coast are double to triple those found on the West Coast. It seems to have been the late British geneticist L. S. Penrose who, in 1957, first theorized that the presence or absence of something in drinking water, a trace metal perhaps, could explain the geographical meandering of neural tube defects. Since then, analyzing local water supplies and local rates of spina bifida and anencephaly has become almost a separate branch of epidemiology. Researchers have studiously pored over United States water-quality reports; they have descended on the coal-mining valleys of Wales—which have a high rate of neural tube deformities—and they have drawn and collated water in taps from Glasgow to Vancouver.

Although not every study concurs, basically this twenty-year pursuit of drinking water has settled on the question of water hardness—the combined concentration of magnesium and calcium. With impressive regularity, there has been a "negative correlation" between water hardness and neural tube defects—in effect, the higher the magnesium and calcium content, the smaller the number of local children who are malformed. In the United States, the mean water hardness of the states with substantial spina bifida is 88 ppm (parts per million); in states with little spina bifida, it is 157 ppm. In thirty-six Canadian cities surveyed, infant deaths from anencephaly tended to fall as water calcium levels rose; and, similarly, in forty-eight localities in South Wales, the prevalence of congenital malformations at birth was observed to fall as local water hardness increased.

The fact of negative correlation, however, says nothing about the why. As there is no reason to think that a higher amount of calcium or magnesium per se in the mother's drinking water protects fetal brain development, a secondary or synergistic association was sought to explain these data. The trouble is that drinking water, with its huge load of both natural and human-made chemicals, presents secondary associations without number. "Soft waters," Jean Fedrick, an Oxford University epidemiologist, once pointed out in *Nature*, "are more likely to dissolve metals from pipes through which they pass . . . or, alternatively, a mild teratogenic agent added to, or already in, the water might be inactivated by the calcium . . . [or] it could be that a part is played by the deficiency of calcium in soft water, although the amounts of calcium involved would make this unlikely." Or it might be that high levels of calcium or magnesium cause more spontaneous abortions; with malformed fetuses generally being the first to abort, the appearance of fewer malformations at birth in hard water areas would, in that case, be a statistical tease.

It has proven impossible to wade through all these variables to reach a conclusion. Like any other endeavor, medical research has its bottom line. The bottom line for the saga of neural tube defects is that two decades of pursuing this association have yielded more measurements of water hardness than anyone knows what to do with, and not one solid clue to preventing anencephaly, spina bifida, or hydrocephaly. Literally hundreds of efforts to establish environmental causes for Down's syndrome, limb reduction deformities, cleft palates, and other major malformations have ended in a similar impasse. Not surprisingly, the balance in time and money against teratogens discovered began to cause disenchantment with the search. In the early 1970s, the wheel turned a few degrees and some people suggested that either it was time to concede that most congenital malformations "may just be the survivors of a continuous supply of mutations which are (and have been throughout time) randomly produced to allow the species to adjust to the ecosystem," or that, even allowing a major environmental role in malformation, "in that fine and private place, the womb, the environmental influences at work are likely to remain obscure and unpredictable accidents . . . due, in part, perhaps, to minor disturbances of delicately balanced maternal metabolic factors beyond our control."

Actually, the most important thing that had come from this thirty-year preoccupation with teratogenesis was simply an appreciation of how vulnerable, and yet how paradoxically tough, the human embryo is. As a convention, people speak of the first trimester of pregnancy as the danger period for malformations, but closer study has taught that the real span of danger is even shorter. During the first week following fertilization, when the embryo, then technically known as a blastocyst, lies free within the uterus, environmental agents may possibly kill it, but malformations compatible with live birth do not seem to occur. The periods of tissue differentiation and organogenesis (organ formation), which are the true periods of susceptibility to teratogens, begin at about day eighteen, more than a week after the embryo first starts attaching to the uterine wall. Organogenesis is completed by the eighth week, or fifty-sixth day, post-fertilization. The embryo, then barely an inch long, is basically formed. During the remainder of gestation, or the fetal period, toxins may still exact a high toll on the growing being—they may, for example, blind, cause mental retardation, or injure the external sex organs—but having achieved eight weeks and an inch, the embryo is safe from major structural malformations. This quickly gained safety makes it all the more breathcatching that, only weeks or days earlier, a very small dose of a common tranquilizing agent such as thalidomide could have so consummately destroyed limbs and structure; it also makes it all the more frustrating that science, with all its tools, laboratory equipment, computers, and epidemiological forays, has so little idea of how to accomplish the task of protecting a one-inch embryo for a mere two months.

As so often occurs, however, just as the frustration reached its height, another way of looking at things seemed to offer a breakthrough of sorts. Since about 1976, some epidemiologists have simply tried to identify places with birth-defect clusters; they have found that, among other places, the environs of airports, chemical dumps, and some factory complexes are places where unusual numbers of malformed children may be born. Since dozens of toxic chemicals may leak from dumps or spew from factories, this approach may never manage to specify the precise ones responsible. Still, the "geographical" approach to birth defects has suggested environmental links that were previously obscure; it does give us some idea where we stand. To Peter Infante, a young epidemiologist with the National Institute of Occupational Safety and Health, "It would not be surprising that you could draw up a birth defects map of the United States, in much the same way that the National Cancer Institute has published an atlas of deaths by locality, which would show a concentration of defects in areas with certain environmental influences." Dr. Infante's own special interest is the reproductive hazards of vinyl chloride. He has reported that the incidence of neural tube malformations is unusually high in some towns with polyvinyl-chloride factories; he has also reported that the pregnancies of the wives of workers who deal with the gaseous vinyl-chloride monomer—but not solidified polyvinyl chloride—end in an unusual number of fetal deaths. Since the vinyl-chloride monomer is a well-documented mutagen in test systems, these fetal deaths might well reflect lethal mutations to the sperm of the fathers.

Whether birth defects and geography will turn out to be consistently clear-cut is something other people tend to doubt. Still, the number of local situations that, in a few years' time, have been documented throughout the United States and in other countries are beginning to add up—and they suggest that many birth defects, which might otherwise be dismissed as "unpredictable accidents," are really about as accidental as a sledgehammer.

Just off Route 62 in the city of Niagara Falls, New York, and just a few feet after Luck Avenue changes into Colvin Boulevard, there is a chain-link fence, put there by the state, which guards three blocks of evacuated homes where a vision of industrialism came to a shattering end. In the late 1890s, an entrepreneur named William T. Love started to build a "model" industrial city in the area. He planned for it to be home to 600,000 workers and appropriate factories for them to work in. Love went bankrupt on this dream, and about the only substantial thing he left behind was a partially dug section of canal, through which he had intended to connect the upper and lower levels of the Niagara River, to provide his model community with immense waterpower. In the 1920s, this ditch became a disposal site for the toxic wastes of several chemical companies. In 1953, the Hooker Chemicals and Plastics Corporation, which owned the site, covered it over and sold it to the city for a token $1; it was used by the Board of Education as an elementary school site, and, in the late 1950s, developers erected about a hundred modest but comfortable homes right along the landfill's edge. In 1976, after abnormally heavy rains, leakage from the thousands of drums of buried chemicals came "percolating to the surface." It spilled into the yards and basements of nearby homes and into the playground of the elementary school, where, according to residents, it literally "swallowed" the third base of the children's baseball field. By 1978, when the New York State Department of Health proposed evacuating all those residents whose homes immediately bordered the canal, the remnant of Love's dream was nationally known as the Love Canal Disaster.

Even before the heavy rains brought the chemicals into sight and smell, residents of the area believed something was wrong. Animals kept as pets often died prematurely, and cancer deaths among the human population seemed out of hand. Toward the end of 1978, however, when the State Department of Health published its findings of a house-by-house survey, children, once again, stood out as the primary victims of "chemical percolation." Conceiving and trying to bear children in an area where the air level of some toxic chemicals measured 250 to 5,000 times above their established safety levels were problematic in themselves. In the Ninety-ninth Street south area directly bordering the canal, depending on their age group, women were experiencing almost double to three-and-a-half times the generally expected number of spontaneous abortions. And, among twenty-four living children on this block, there were four with severe birth defects. One little girl was born with slight retardation, a cleft palate, and later grew an extra row of bottom teeth. Children living in the vicinity of the canal also suffered from a range of other problems, including hearing defects, respiratory difficulties, and urinary blockages, which may or may not be permanent. Since leaving the area, one deaf boy is said to have regained his hearing, and a little girl, so severely retarded in growth that doctors had told her parents to expect that she might well be a midget, has begun to gain weight and grow rapidly.

By the end of 1978, New York State had decided that the risks of having people live near the Love Canal were insupportable. For $7.4 million, it bought the homes of 237 families in the immediate area, evacuated them, and closed off the site with a fence. The fence, however, hardly marked the final chapter of the Love Canal Disaster. Dr. Beverly Paigen, a biologist at Roswell Park Memorial Institute, a major research center in Buffalo, New York, has continued to investigate the health of families left behind and living from one to five blocks from the canal. Their lot, in many cases, seems as dismal as that of the evacuated families, the apparent reason being that old streambeds, which crisscrossed the canal, have spread the chemicals farther than first thought.

In the past five years, nine of sixteen children born to families living along these old streambeds had birth defects; these include one child who was born with three ears. Women of childbearing age who had happened to move to homes along the streambeds had triple the number of miscarriages they had formerly experienced. And, in a preliminary survey of convulsive disorders, Dr. Paigen learned that there were twice as many epileptics living in homes along the streambeds as even living in the "dry" parts of the unevacuated canal area. Five of these epileptics were children—one nineteen-year-old who has now gone away to college has noticed a real lessening in the intensity of his seizures. In February 1979, in recognition of the increasingly bad news, the state urged pregnant women and families with children under two years of age within a twenty-block radius around the canal to get out. It is not apparent, however, just how they are to go about getting out, since the state is not willing to buy more homes in the area, and many of these families lack the funds to start life again on their own.

The federal Environmental Protection Agency now estimates that there are about 2,500 similar toxic landfills and open dumps scattered across the United States, and that perhaps eight hundred of these pose as serious a health threat as the Love Canal—either potentially or, perhaps, at the present moment. As other states begin to contend with their industrial waste sites, will their health departments find as many deaf and retarded and malformed children as were found near the ditch William Love left behind?

In counterpoint to the Love Canal and its tale of teratogenic (or mutagenic, or a combination of the two) danger in buried wastes, other recent work has suggested the similar danger of things that drift from the sky. A few years before the Love Canal became a headline, Dr. F. Nowell Jones, a psychologist at the University of California at Los Angeles, had become intrigued with reports suggesting an unusual rate of mental disturbance among people who lived close to airports. As he began to look into "airport health," Dr. Jones found something that intrigued him even more—birth defects in the vicinity of airports. In 1978, after analyzing more than 225,000 births over a three-year period, he showed that babies born to parents who lived partly or wholly within the approach pattern of Los Angeles International Airport had a defects rate of almost twelve per thousand births; in the remainder of Los Angeles County, the rate was seven per thousand births. The increase in defects among these children covered a wide spectrum of abnormalities. There were more children with, among other things, anencephaly, spina bifida, harelip, and cleft palate. This initial birth-defects report, of course, needs confirmation; but previous reports of excessive stillbirths in the environs of London's Heathrow Airport and of low-birthweight babies born near Osaka Airport in Japan certainly support the impression that airports are an adverse prenatal environment.

In the intense discussion surrounding possible causes for the pregnancy problems near airports, suspicion has primarily focused on noise and fuel pollution. But Dr. Milton Zaret, the ophthalmologist known for his theory about the role of microwaves in heart attacks, has also pointed out that "most busy airports are richly endowed with electronic smog emanating from radar, navigation, radio and telecommunications networks, as well as from high-power electronic transmission lines." Dr. Zaret thought this electronic smog was also worth investigating.

Dr. Jones personally favors noise as the most likely suspect. He has pointed out both that loud noises were long ago shown to be a stress on the mother that could provoke gross abnormalities in fetal mice and rats, and that the noise level in homes around Los Angeles Airport reaches to a hundred times that of an ordinary suburban residence. He doubts that electronic smog or, by implication, microwaves, are reaching these homes in high enough levels to cause birth defects. Actually, he considers the idea "nonsense."

On the other hand, another doctor not long ago found an unusual cluster of birth defects and immediately suspected radar—meaning microwaves—as the cause. In 1972, Dr. Peter B. Peacock, then chairman of the Department of Public Health and Epidemiology at the University of Alabama, learned that about four times the "normal" number of children with clubfoot had been born at the Lyster Army Hospital in Fort Rucker in the previous year and a half. There were seventeen clubfooted children in all, as well as an unusual number of children with cleft palate and other abnormalities.

Fort Rucker is a military aviation center with forty-eight radar installations located within a thirty-mile radius of it—facts that seemed to point toward microwaves like an accusatory finger. But, as recounted in *The Zapping of America*, Paul Brodeur's exhaustive investigation of microwave pollution, Dr. Peacock was never able to proceed very far with his suspicions. The Army declined to give him access to these children's medical records, their parents' employment histories, and other information required for a proper study. Nonetheless, after a few years of futile tilting with the Army, Dr. Peacock did come across some corroborating evidence for a microwave connection. He learned that the fathers of all seventeen of the clubfooted children were helicopter pilots; because much of their flying is done at very low altitudes, helicopter pilots are constantly exposed to the "electronic smog" that hovers over the airports, and therefore sustain far greater microwave doses than either airplane pilots or ground personnel.

The situation in North Karelia, Finland, has also contributed to suspicions about microwaves. In early 1977, to considerable relief, the Finnish government announced that a five-year program to deal with the strange heart attack problem in its eastern provinces was working very well. In North Karelia, once the scene of the world's highest rate of heart attack, as the government had prodded people to give up their cigarettes, eat less fat, and seek treatment for hypertension, the male heart attack rate had dropped by 40 percent. This was a major achievement, and, of course, not one encouraging of Zaret's microwave theory; on the other hand, the ophthalmologist had only proposed microwaves as a contributing factor to the Finnish dilemma, not the sole cause.

This five-year no-smoking, low-fat program, did not, however, address something else distinctive about North Karelia— namely, its high birth-defect rate. Anencephaly and cleft palate, for example, are two defects on which the Finns keep close tabs as possible indicators of an environmental problem, and the rate of both in North Karelia is almost double the Finnish average. The Finnish rate for cleft palate especially, in the one-word summary of Irma Saxen, of the Department of Pathology at the University of Helsinki, is "conspicuous." She adds, "It is probably the highest reported for Caucasoid populations." Without North Karelia, however, the national Finnish average stands at a respectable 0.87 per 1,000 live births. North Karelia stands conspicuously off by itself with 1.47 per 1,000 live births.

Finnish epidemiologists have pointed out that, in North Karelia, with its farming and country traditions, women still tend to have more children and keep having them later in life than in the rest of Finland. But whether this really accounts for the birth-defects rate there is something no one has closely analyzed. It

might also be of use if the Finnish government, or the World
Health Organization, which was much concerned about the heart
attacks in North Karelia, took some microwave readings in the
area.

Knowing the powers of the technological devices in use
today—one is reminded that the radar across the lake from North
Karelia is sending signals to Iowa and back—it would probably
surprise no one to learn that we had entered an era where other
countries can literally blast out the brains of fetuses across their
borders. Even the possibility adds a blunt urgency to the epidemiological task of identifying teratogens. In this brave new world,
it is ever more imperative not to make mistakes about the
teratogenicity of agents in common use. What chance is there of
really working through the variables of a situation like the Love
Canal, where eighty-two toxic chemicals have been identified
among the seeping wastes; or that of Los Angeles Airport, where
noise, radar, and fuel exhaust all have some claims of being
dangerous to the fetus; or that of industrial communities, where
any number of factories might be suspected of contributing to
local birth defects?

Although past experience with epidemiology shows it is not
easy to answer these questions, a few brilliant exceptions have
broken through the impasse—exceptions that throw a perspective
on the strange blend of luck, insight, and persistence needed to see
the danger sometimes lurking in familiar things. Ironically, where
looking at the big, geographical picture had, once again, focused
attention on the environment, looking at things in a very small,
tidy way emerged as an effective means of flushing out individual
teratogens.

That alcohol may injure unborn children had sufficiently
impressed itself on the ancient world to influence both myth and
custom. Vulcan, the blacksmith of the Roman gods, was said to
have been born lame because his father, Jupiter, conceived him

while drunk. In Sparta and Carthage, as a protection against the birth of deformed children, bridal couples were forbidden to drink on their wedding night. In the eighteenth century, British pamphleteers, among them Henry Fielding, wrote flaming tracts about the dangers of alcohol to unborn children, and in 1726 the College of Physicians petitioned the Parliament to control the distillation of cheap gin, condemning the stuff as "a cause of weak, feeble, distempered children." In the nineteenth century, American evangelists and prohibitionists took up a similar theme—although their way of stating their concern was somewhat lurid. One evangelist spoke of "the depravity stamped, like the mark of Cain, upon the foreheads of the posterity of drunken parents."

Of course, neither the ancient Spartans nor American evangelists understood the principles of teratology. Theirs was just an instinctive belief that the sorry condition of the offspring of alcoholics somehow reflected the liquor consumption of the parents. Twentieth-century science considered itself too rational to pay attention to these several centuries of observation. In their 1940 book, *Alcohol Explored,* Howard W. Haggard and E. M. Jellinek, both members of the Research Council on the Problems of Alcohol, derided "the efforts of those investigators who have tried to gather evidence of the birth of idiots and other types of defective children conceived while the parents were said to be in a state of intoxification. Such spectacular studies do not yield valid evidence," they grumbled. "They belong more in the realm of rumormongering than in that of scientific study." By the early 1970s, about all that had been scientifically conceded was that maternal alcoholism could impair the physical and developmental growth of the child. (In 1968, as it happens, a French researcher did issue detailed descriptions of congenital abnormalities observed in 127 children of alcoholic women. However, as American physicians no more read French medical journals than they trust to pagan myth, the idea of alcohol as a specific teratogen did not then cross the Atlantic.)

The concern of the English-speaking world with the teratogenicity of alcohol began in the early 1970s when a young doctor named Kenneth L. Jones had a fellowship in pediatric dysmorphol-ogy—a specialty focused on the care of malformed children—at the University of Washington in Seattle. A colleague asked him to look over several children born to alcoholic women. Jones had the impression that these children were suffering from a definite syndrome of malformation, characterized mainly by small size, mental retardation, and craniofacial and heart abnormalities. His observations were published in *Lancet* in June 1973, with the syndrome having been given the name "Fetal Alcohol Syn-drome"—or, for short, FAS. Since the Jones team had found defects among the children of white, black, and Indian alcoholics alike, it seemed unlikely a genetic condition was at fault; and since the mothers included some who were exclusively addicted to wine or beer or spirits, it was also unlikely the fault lay with an additive to a specific fermentation process. Alcohol, itself, has been accepted as the basic problem—although, perhaps, a problem augmented by the malnourishment and poor health of alcoholic mothers.

Although the idea of alcohol as a teratogen is now well documented, not all observers have found that the defects to the children comprise a specific syndrome. Four years later, for example, a group of Massachusetts physicians reported in the *New England Journal of Medicine* that infants born to a group of "heavy drinkers" who had delivered at Boston City Hospital had double the malformation rate of infants born to "moderate" drinkers—but "a specific pattern of anomalies was not noticed." These Boston children were also closely tested for signs of neurological damage; the children of heavy drinkers tended to be very jittery and many of them were not able to suck their formula well. Something positive that came out of the Boston study, however, was evidence that no small number of alcoholic mothers can manage to give up drinking during their pregnancies. Boston City Hospital now includes alcoholic treatment among its prenatal services. In the group reported on, one third of the heavy drinkers substantially reduced their alcoholic intake. The general well-being of children born to them was about the same as that for the ordinary run of children delivered at Boston Hospital—a place where it is "normal," in any case, for 35 percent of newborns to appear in a condition that requires their being placed in intensive care.

The quandary now is to determine the levels of alcohol consumption that injure unborn children. The women Dr. Jones first studied were chronic alcoholics, "in such bad shape," he recalls, "that many had the DT's." The "heavy" drinkers in Boston, with their large number of malformed children, consumed an average of 174 milliliters (almost 6 ounces) of "absolute alcohol" a day—absolute alcohol being 100 percent pure alcohol; in more familiar terms, they would have been drinking about six stiff drinks or a couple of bottles of wine daily. Evidently, alcohol is not a one-dose teratogen as was thalidomide. Millions of women have had an occasional drink, or even several drinks, while pregnant without visible harm to their children.

Below some indistinct level of consumption, and past the first months of pregnancy, however, liquor would no longer announce its impact in visible deformities. "Then," comments Dr. Jones, "you are talking about the effect on the growth of cells, particularly brain cells." Many people now believe the amount of alcohol that may interfere with body and brain growth to be rather small. Dr. Sergio Fabro, the chief of Fetal–Maternal Medicine at George Washington University, has offered what he calls "the intelligent guess that substantial and serious risk may begin with the consumption of three ounces of absolute alcohol a day." One investigator has reported that infants whose mothers drank just one ounce of absolute alcohol daily during the last half of pregnancy weigh about one-third pound less at birth than do the newborns of abstinent women. In itself, this is not drastic; but low weight at birth is sometimes a signal of a permanent growth deficit. The infants of smokers are another group who tend to be underweight when born, and follow-up in later years has shown them to be just slightly shorter than their peers and slightly behind in their achievement at school.

*

Five years before Dr. Jones described his first group of alcohol-injured children, a small report in a Russian medical journal signaled the discovery of a teratogen that would be, if anything, more startling than that of alcohol. The Russians told of thirty-one pregnancies among anesthesiologists—fully two thirds of which had come to greater or lesser grief. Eighteen of the anesthesiologists lost their children to spontaneous abortions, two went into premature labor, and one gave birth to a malformed child. In the following years, alerted by the Russian signal, other people began to look at the pregnancy experiences of women occupationally exposed to anesthesia, and the reports came in like bullets from an international six-shooter, emptying their observations in loud, angry reports from around the globe. The Danes, English, and Americans alike reported that women who worked in operating rooms were experiencing up to triple the miscarriage rate of other female hospital personnel; and they had more malformed children. It was, of course, not reassuring of the general state of environmental awareness that the medical profession had long failed to perceive this pregnancy carnage in its own ranks.

In 1842, Dr. Crawford Long of Jefferson County, Georgia, applied ether to a friend and performed the world's first operation under a general anesthetic. For his trouble, Long was run out of town by Jefferson County residents who believed him in league with the devil. No doubt part of the reason anesthesia so long escaped ordinary investigations and suspicions about its toxicity was that the medical profession regarded it with almost the same awe as did Jefferson County—except that, for doctors, anesthesia was a discovery in the miracle class. The public, too, came to understand that it was "one of America's greatest contributions to the world." But anesthesia's escape from questioning was more than a miracle might fairly claim for itself; it reflected the stubborn, almost irrational immunity that the medical profession accords its own favored devices and tools. Apparently, no one seems to have even thought to run major surgical anesthetics such as halothane, methoxyflurane, and nitrous oxide through a few pregnant rats until the 1960s. And even after the Russians, English, and Danes had revealed the pregnancy problems of their operating-room workers, critics of anesthesia were not welcomed by their colleagues. In 1974, a young anesthesiologist named Thomas Corbett decided to animal-test isoflurane, a new anesthetic the FDA had almost made up its mind to approve, for possible harm to the fetus—testing the FDA had never required. Dr. Corbett's paper, describing later liver and uterine tumors in mice exposed to isoflurane as fetuses and infants, was accepted for publication in *Anesthesia and Analgesia,* the official journal of the International Anesthesia Research Society; but it was never printed.

Nonetheless, enough research has been done—and enough printed—to gain quite a clear picture of the reproductive hazards of anesthesia. The American Society of Anesthesiologists has, by now, surveyed virtually all persons in the United States who work in operating rooms—this includes the full membership of the ASA itself, of the American Association of Nurse Anesthetists, the American Association of Operating Room Technicians, and the American Association of Operating Room Nurses—and reported on the health of the 50,000 people who responded to its questionnaire. Not unexpectedly, the ASA found that the reproductive health of female operating-room employees was grim. Nurses who worked in operating rooms had a 60 percent higher rate of deformed children than nurses who worked elsewhere in hospitals; female anesthesiologists had twice the rate of malformed children of other female physicians.

The ASA survey was also the first to question male operating-room personnel about the health of their children. Fully 25 percent more male anesthesiologists said their children had major malformations—these included children with conditions such as spina bifida, abnormal hearts, and cleft palates—than did male physicians who did not deal with anesthesia. To the ASA, this was "an unexpected finding [that] represents a matter for serious concern and deserves further investigation." The concern, of course, was that anesthesia was a mutagen. Like the clubfooted youngsters of helicopter pilots in Alabama and the fetal deaths linked to vinyl chloride, the malformed children of these male anesthesiologists served as a reminder that "it takes two gametes to make a zygote."

Further investigation, however, has not really settled whether anesthesia does mutate sperm—the male gamete. The British have since investigated the rate of malformation among children of more than five thousand male physicians. They found, rather ambiguously, that those born to doctors who worked in operating rooms had more minor, but not more major, abnormalities than those born to other doctors. In the United States, a slight excess of malformations has also since been found among the children of male dental surgeons—again, an ambiguous result. What is not ambiguous is that the miscarriage rate of female dental surgeons almost approaches that of female anesthesiologists; these women would appear to be yet another group at high risk from anesthesia.

Making operating rooms safer for the people who work there, and perhaps for their children, has turned out to be devastatingly simple. For $100 or less, most anesthesia machines can be equipped with "scavenging hoses," which capture about 90 percent of the waste gas otherwise allowed to escape into the operating room. People in the field seem confident that scavenging is the answer to reducing, if not fully ending, the pregnancy and other health problems, including high rates of cancer, that seem to plague operating-room personnel. The ASA has promised to undertake a similar survey of "scavenged" operating rooms. Should that survey confirm everyone's hopes of improvement, it will be an encouraging environmental lesson—but also a lesson that contains the bitter knowledge that hundreds of children were, for the want of a little perception and $100, injured for life. For some physicians, the official recognition that operating-room workers have difficult and often disastrous pregnancies has been like having a subconscious note brought to blaring attention. One doctor, for instance, remembers a very kindly obstetrician at the hospital where she spent her residency. Many of the nurses and other doctors at the hospital chose him to deliver their own babies.

"He pulled out one malformed baby after another," she recalls. "I think he started to believe it was his own fault somehow. I heard he began to go on terrible drinking binges. Now I wonder to what extent anesthesia explains those children."

The damage to unborn children from alcohol and from anesthesia had first come to attention by looking at small groups— but groups selected for a known exposure to a less than benign substance. The value of looking at small, selected groups also held for the third teratogenic agent identified at about this time.

In early 1972, Dr. Audrey Nora and Dr. James Nora, a husband-and-wife team of pediatricians then practicing in Denver, Colorado, happened to observe, on the same day in two different hospitals, two newborns with drastic deformities somewhat reminiscent of the worst wreckage of thalidomide. The normal rate of such multiple deformities is probably less than one in 50,000 live births. "We were really bothered by these two children," James Nora recalls, "so we decided to collect some background information on them and also on some other, similar children we were able to locate."

Their background search led the Noras to a very disconcerting conclusion. Sex hormones were the single suspect compound to which these badly deformed children had most frequently been exposed as fetuses. Almost simultaneously, however, other researchers were finding a similar background of sex hormone exposure in children with heart defects, limb reduction deformities, and certain other malformations. For the most part, exposure to the hormones had occurred in the now notorious form of "pregnancy supports" and the now discredited form of hormonal pregnancy tests. Sometimes the exposure occurred when the women had "breakthrough" pregnancies while on birth control pills, or had taken pills without realizing they were already pregnant. The long era of hormone use during pregnancy was about to come to a tottering end—an end that even the discovery of cancer among children exposed to DES had not been able to bring about. (When DES was censured in 1971, many physicians just turned to other hormone preparations for their pregnant patients.)

The Noras later proposed the acronym VACTERL (*v*ertebral, *a*nal, *c*ardiac, *t*racheo*e*sophageal, *r*enal, and *l*imb) for the devastating pattern of multiple deformities they believe can sometimes follow prenatal exposure to sex hormones. Like the Fetal Alcohol Syndrome, the idea of a specific syndrome of hormone-caused deformity is still argued in medicine; that prescribed sex hormones badly, and sometimes fatally, injure a child is, however, no longer much argued in itself. More than a half-dozen studies, concerning a variety of malformations, have now testified to this point. The evidence is especially strong for a hormone link to heart deformities—of a sort that often kill—and to limb reduction deformities. In 1974, moreover, Dr. Dwight Janerich of the New York State Birth Defects Institute pointed out that the rate of limb reduction deformities among New York State children during the previous decade had climbed from 0.15 to 0.20 per 1,000 births. These numbers represented a 33 percent increase in the ranks of children who will, say, spend their lives confined to wheelchairs, or on crutches, or picking up things with orthopedic claws instead of their own hands. During almost the same period, the Canadian provinces of Alberta and British Columbia experienced an even larger increase in limb reduction deformities. All told, Dr. Samuel Shapiro, co-director of the Boston University Drug Epidemiology Unit, testified in 1978 to the Select Committee on Population of the House of Representatives, "There are reasonable grounds to suspect that female hormones cause cardiac deformities, and perhaps other major deformities as well."

Even though this general conclusion had been reached, the era of hormone supports during pregnancy had not come to a complete end. Actually, the FDA had "withdrawn approval" for the pregnancy-related use of progestational hormones—including those sold under the brand names Provera, Depo-Provera, Delalutin, Duphaston, Norlutin, and Norlutate—by early 1974. And to underline its "disapproval" of prescribing such agents during pregnancy, the FDA penned yet another emphatic warning on the subject in its January–March Drug Bulletin of 1975—a bulletin sent to every practicing physician in the nation, and said to be read by most of them. "FDA emphasizes," began this warning, "that estrogenic and progestational hormones should not be used in early pregnancy for any purpose. Such use of these sex hormones may seriously damage the fetus (congenital anomalies, including heart and limb reduction defects)."

This warning was to little purpose. Like the estrogen preparations used as pregnancy supports, most of these progestational hormones have remained on the market because they have other uses. (Depo-Provera, for instance, is used to treat certain advanced cancers.) Freely available as they are, physicians continued to prescribe them freely. The Health Research Group has reported that, in 1975, American doctors wrote 533,000 prescriptions for hormone use during pregnancy. The stated "indications" ranged from "to prevent miscarriage" to the more nebulous "prenatal care"—but, in any case, all were uses disapproved by the FDA.

The 1975 figures, which came from a private marketing research firm, have apparently not been publicly updated. Still, virtually no one believes that hormone use in pregnancy is under full control even yet. One government official very concerned about these matters says that, from his own conversations with Washington-area obstetricians, he would "not be surprised" to learn that, in 1979, hormones were still being prescribed for 5 percent or more of pregnant women in the area. Hormone supports, apparently, are a rather fashionable therapy in the nation's capital—and, among physicians and patients alike, a lot of this sort of prescribing does have to do with what is fashionable. Even careful doctors are finding it hard to contend with women who remain convinced that hormone supports are a magic antidote for pregnancy problems or threatened miscarriage. "Some really press you to prescribe them," comments a New York doctor. "I won't prescribe sex hormones for this purpose myself, but I know that many patients who are worried about a miscarriage will go from doctor to doctor until they find someone who will give them hormones. And they do always find someone."

Hormonal pregnancy supports comprise both an incredible chapter in medical history and a chapter that remains incredibly veiled. Except for the interest in the cancer of the DES daughters, both the medical profession and the public alike seem to have failed substantially to understand what happened. Although, for example, medical researchers may not agree that there is a specific fetal alcohol syndrome, only a few years after the recognition of the teratogenicity of alcohol, research reports generally concur that a "malformation rate" of around 30 percent is common among the children of alcoholic mothers. Twenty years after the first reports of progestin-caused pseudohermaphroditism, medical research still has no clear notion of even the range of defects caused by pregnancy supports and virtually no notion at all of the true rate of malformation associated with the use of these preparations. While the available evidence does suggest that the overall rate is rather low, since they were used as hormone supports for two decades and in millions of pregnancies, by now they may well have disfigured as many children as thalidomide did—not to mention that, unlike thalidomide, they also contain a cancer risk. But there is not the public shock there was over thalidomide. It may be that the human mind only has room for one birth-defects disaster, one Watergate, and one Vietnam every generation. Attention wanders.

The United States was not the sole place where sex hormones remained in use despite many warnings. In 1975, for instance, the same year that American doctors wrote more than 500,000 prescriptions for hormones during pregnancy, the Hadassah Hospital Medical School reported that fully 19 percent of pregnant women in West Jerusalem had "been given therapeutic hormones during pregnancy." The Israelis had followed the American lead here as they often do in other matters. Today they are seeking other advice: they have asked some of the American women organizing self-help and support groups for DES families to help them in the sad chore of organizing their own DES population.

*

When James Wilson wrote that the cause of 65 to 70 percent of birth defects was unknown, it was 1973. At the time, the traditional epidemiological effort to painstakingly link one type of malformation to one cause was at a stalemate. Yet, by 1979, by looking at things somewhat differently—by taking the geography of malformation or beginning with suspicious agents and small groups—researchers had managed to suggest environmental causes for substantial numbers of defects. No one has yet attempted to add up these "geographical and agent" observations— and some are still tentative—but, all told, they would seem to represent substantial insights into preventing much harm and human misery.

In a sense, however, for all their importance to individual lives, the questions these breakthroughs and insights left behind were almost larger than the questions they answered. Why, for example, are hormones evidently teratogenic after brief use, while the teratogenicity of alcohol seems to depend on chronic use? On the other hand, why are perhaps 30 percent of the children of alcoholic, or "heavy drinking," mothers born with congenital malformations, while even the daily use of hormone supports seems to elicit relatively few serious malformations? After all the investigations of operating rooms, alcohol, and hormones, the hows and whys of birth defects remained as elusive as ever. Scientists still could go no further than the exasperated statement of a government scientist that most defects were probably "the result of teratogenic agents acting on susceptible individuals by mechanisms known only to God."

Leaving behind the world of gross structural damage for the less visible metabolic, functional, and behavioral injuries, however, researchers no longer found themselves so often trudging down a muddied, inconclusive trail, like spies left out in the cold.

In just a few years of concentrated work on this question, evidence for environmental links to "subtler" defects, such as brain damage and growth retardation, has piled up fast.

The reason for the research success is a frank loss to society. Lesser damage to the fetus is now widespread enough that it can often be readily documented. Some agents are almost breathtaking in the precision of their targets: they will bypass the whole child only to interfere with blood coagulation, or bile metabolism, or dig into a specific region of the brain. Others just seem to stifle growth generally: in lay language, infants who have come under their influence would be called "puny"; in pediatric language, these infants are described as "failing to thrive."

Cigarette smoking, the premier example of an agent that stifles growth, is perhaps the single most studied toxic influence on pregnancy. The first hint of harm from cigarettes came in 1957 when Dr. Wina J. Simpson, a public health specialist in San Bernadino, California, reported that women who smoked had almost double the number of premature children as nonsmoking mothers. The hardcore estimate of the cigarette toll came in 1974 when the United States Surgeon General estimated that smoking was directly responsible for 5 percent of American perinatal deaths, those being deaths that occur between twenty weeks' gestation and one week after birth. Between these observations, cigarette smoking and pregnancy outcome have been the focus of some forty-five studies, covering a half-million pregnancies worldwide. They tell an almost uniformly dismal tale of miscarriages, complications, and infant deaths. A series from the Johns Hopkins University School of Public Health, based on the outcome of more than fifty thousand pregnancies and published in three parts over five years, commands special attention for the insights it provides both into the clinical management of smokers' pregnancies and the mechanisms of damage from smoking.

"What we did," explains Mary Meyer, the associate professor of epidemiology who led this giant effort, "was to first show there was a relationship between smoking and perinatal death. Then, we were interested in the biological reasons for the relationship. And finally, we looked for clinical signs common to smokers' pregnancies, which could alert a physician to later trouble. Obviously, not all women who smoke experience pregnancy complications, but one thing we found which obstetricians should know about is that bleeding before twenty weeks was closely correlated with early neonatal deaths, or those in the first week after birth. So, an obstetrician confronted with a patient with early bleeding in pregnancy would be well-advised to make sure she wasn't a smoker."

In brief outline, the Meyer team first concluded that "the risk of perinatal death increased directly with the smoking level"—by 22 percent when a mother smoked less than a pack a day, and by 44 percent when a mother smoked more than a pack a day. The Meyer team next learned that mothers who had smoked had more low-birthweight children (infants who weigh less than 2,500 grams, or 5 pounds 8 ounces) and more preterm children (those born before thirty-eight weeks' gestation) than women who didn't smoke. They further observed that smokers' pregnancies had rather a large incidence of placental complications and that, overall, more than one quarter of the smokers' pregnancies that had ended in fetal or neonatal death had lapsed into incidents of vaginal bleeding before twenty weeks' gestation.

Together, these observations drew an incisive portrait of smokers' pregnancies. The observations about placental complications, for example, reached beyond epidemiology to provide a clue for the testing of drugs and chemicals. As Meyer has pointed out, these complications are also common among women who live at high altitudes; they are often the contortions of a placenta struggling for air. Their appearance in smoking mothers makes it probable that carbon monoxide, the component of cigarette smoke that reduces the blood's oxygen-carrying capacity, may be the component most deeply implicated in pregnancy problems; assessing their interference in oxygen transport could serve as a guide to the fetotoxicity of other substances.

In their observations about vaginal bleeding, the Meyer team had, of course, also reached beyond epidemiology to provide doctors and women with an alarm signal that a pregnancy is in severe trouble; and, finally, they showed that the prematurity and birthweight worked together in an interesting way: that is, smokers' babies were not just underweight in general, but underweight because they were not making it to term. "We have shown," Meyer concluded, "that the excess of perinatal mortality associated with maternal smoking is made up of early fetal deaths due to anoxia [oxygen deprivation] or to unknown causes and of neonatal deaths occuring mainly because of premature delivery."

There is some evidence that even women who give up smoking will continue to have troubled pregnancies for some time afterward; there is other evidence that giving up smoking by the fourth month of pregnancy may restore the normal odds of producing a live child. In any event, smoking does not only deal in fetal life or death. It is also one of the few toxic influences on pregnancy that has been followed on a mass scale for "subtle" neurological disorders in the children born. The research implicating prenatal smoking in later hyperactivity and developmental deficits has already been mentioned. In addition, in 1958, the British began a huge followup of several thousand newborns and, looking over these children at age seven and again at age eleven, they learned that the youngsters of women who had smoked more than ten cigarettes a day during the pregnancy were, on average, four months behind in reading ability and about one-half inch shorter than their classmates. Ironically, in a world where people have little choice about the increased number of toxic substances they take in with food, water, and air, cigarettes, which *are* under individual control, remain the agents widely thought to be the single most important toxic influence on pregnancy.

Between 1958 and 1965, the National Institute of Neurological and Communicative Disorders collected detailed information on the background and outcome of 50,282 American pregnancies and then further followed, in detail, the health of thousands of the children until their eighth birthday. Originally, this massive data collection, known as the Collaborative Perinatal Project, was intended to analyze factors that might contribute to neurological disorders, particularly cerebral palsy. Somewhat belatedly, people also realized it was a Fort Knox for studying all types of environmental influences on the fetus. Evidently the largest such collection in the world, it cites, among other things, the mothers' smoking habits, pregnancy complications, socioeconomic background, and employment. It also contains epidemiological information about pregnancy outcome after exposure to any of an enormous sweep of drugs. A major benefit from the Collaborative Perinatal Project has been a 500-page book, *Birth Defects and Drugs in Pregnancy.* Published in 1977, it is the Boston University Hospital Drug Epidemiology Unit's analysis of both the over-the-counter (OTC) and prescription drugs used by the women in this study in relation to malformations in their children.

On the whole, this analysis did not suggest that drugs are a major cause of malformation. There were some suggested associations that seem worth further checking—clubfoot and inguinal hernia, for instance, are two malformations that turned up fairly frequently in association with selected drugs—but not anything as serious as another thalidomide disaster. On the whole, the Drug Epidemiology Unit regarded it as "generally reassuring [there had been] no major epidemic of malformations during the years of recruitment to the study." However, they also noted that the general escape from drug-induced malformations was "more a matter of good fortune than anything else." Not only had the pregnant women in this study population taken dozens and dozens of individual drugs, but the increase in their overall consumption during just the years of the study almost took the breath away. The Boston group found that the percentage of women who used five to ten drugs during pregnancy more than doubled—from 14 percent to 33 percent—during the seven-year span of recruitment to the Perinatal Study, while the portion who used no drugs at all declined from 9 percent to 4 percent. "It is clear," the Boston group gloomily concluded, "that publicity directed to avoiding unnecessary drug use during pregnancy was a failure."

Although the Boston findings suggested that infants were perhaps not paying a major price for this promiscuous drug consumption, questions about nonstructural damage once again caused second thoughts. Aspirin, that ubiquitous, "friendly" wonder drug, is a major case in point. Used medicinally since 1899, and now swallowed in the United States to the tune of nineteen billion tablets a year, aspirin is the drug most commonly taken during pregnancy, as it is throughout life in those nations where people have access to corner drugstores. Although certainly among the most innocuous of medications and one that provides therapeutic value at low risk, aspirin has long been suspect during pregnancy because it is teratogenic to rats. Whether, however, it also causes malformations in the human fetus will probably never be proven or disproven to total satisfaction. Some major studies have found nothing physically amiss with children whose mothers took aspirin in early pregnancy; other studies have discerned a slight increase in malformations—but an increase that could easily be artificial. Studies of aspirin, as of other drugs, invoke what Josef Warkany has termed "the recurring nightmare of deciding whether low rates of malformation are related to treatment or accidental." Women, for example, might self-prescribe aspirin when they are under attack from various viral diseases, including some flu strains, which may injure the fetus in and of themselves.

If not a perfect picture, it was a very reassuring one until, like rock through plate glass, there came some belated realizations that aspirin may uniquely interfere in the biochemistry of pregnancy—first, by interfering with the platelets, the small, cellular bodies that plug internal tears in the small blood vessels and capillaries; and second, by interfering with the prostaglandins, substances that help regulate the length of both gestation and labor. Because aspirin inhibits platelet clumping, adults who take the maximum recommended dose of twelve tablets daily lose about five milliliters a day of blood, which exits through the bowels. The surprise to researchers is that aspirin persists in fetal blood as long as it does. When women take as few as two aspirin tablets two weeks prior to delivery, testing of the blood of their newborns has shown reduced platelet clumping, and the children themselves may occasionally manifest slight gastrointestinal or other bleeding when they are born.

Whether these effects are serious enough to condemn occasional aspirin use in late pregnancy is something that most observers seem to doubt. Dr. Robert Breckenridge of the University of Rochester School of Medicine, and a co-participant in these inquiries, comments that "it's quite clear the platelets didn't work properly in the laboratory, but it is not clear the platelets don't work properly in the kids. The bleeding we did see in a few cases was transitory and stopped by itself. You couldn't make much of it. On the other hand, many women have told me they wouldn't have made it through labor without a few aspirin."

Constant use of aspirin in late pregnancy, however, is another matter. The most condemnatory report on aspirin has come from the Women's Hospital of Sydney, Australia, where in 1975 it was found that four out of sixty-four pregnancies of women who had taken between two and twelve doses of aspirin a day ended in stillbirth. These mothers had a very high rate of anemia—presumably a reflection of aspirin-related blood loss—and they tended both to deliver their children postmaturely and to have long labors. A New York–Cornell University study similarly found that the labor of women who had routinely consumed large amounts of aspirin lasted five hours longer on average than the labor of those who had not.

One might question whether the problem really lies in aspirin itself, or in the standard labeling, which now encourages people to take up to twelve tablets a day without qualification. The Boston Drug Epidemiology Unit investigated pregnancy outcome in women who took aspirin at the lesser and, no doubt more common, intake level of "at least eight days per lunar month." There was no excess of stillbirths or low-birthweight children in this population. Even during pregnancy, for some women—say, those with arthritis or migraine headaches—constant use of aspirin may represent the least risky antidote to pain. For the general population, however, pregnancy is not a time to routinely consume aspirin at the doses now recommended on labels. In 1977, the Food and Drug Advisory Panel on the Review of Internal Analgesics, one of seventeen FDA panels now inquiring into the safety of the vast over-the-counter drug market, did conclude that taking aspirin in late pregnancy could prolong gestation and bleeding; it recommended that product labeling be revised to read that aspirin should not be taken "during the last three months of pregnancy except under the advice and supervision of a physician." This recommendation is now wending its way through the ranks of the FDA.

Meanwhile, two things stand out about the recent insights into aspirin's biochemistry. They are, first, a sturdy reminder that pregnancy is a special condition when even something as admirable as aspirin may abruptly turn ominous. And, second, they remind that very few drugs have been studied at all for their biochemical, as distinct from their teratogenic, impact on pregnancy. This is especially true of the over-the-counter drug market, which, in the Western world, constitutes almost a distinct class of environmental agents—agents, moreover, that are heavily advertised and promiscuously consumed. People tend to think of them as "perfectly safe" just because they are freely available; but there is no reason to think that time won't bring more adverse news about the relations of over-the-counter products to pregnancy.

Finally, it is instructive just to consider the examples of, say, aspirin, alcohol, and cigarettes. They constitute only a small heap in the mass of environmental agents the fetus encounters; yet consider the diverse effects attributed to them: prolonged or curtailed gestation, outright malformation and mental retardation, and an excess of perinatal deaths. They could, among them, hardly have provided a more emphatic rejoinder to the idea that "birth defects" fall into neat patterns. "Disaster," Dr. Robert Miller likes to say, "is just the detectable part of environmental harm."

Slowly I began to apprehend the mighty
difference between the courts of law and
the courts of science. In the one, a man is
prejudged innocent until the body of
proof leaves no alternative other than to
declare him guilty. In the other, a
proposition is prejudged false until a body
of proof leaves no alternative other than
to declare it true.

ROBERT ARDREY
*African Genesis*

# Chapter 3

# PREVENTION, POSSIBLY

About a half-hour drive from downtown Washington, D.C., there
is a shopping center and commercial district known as Tyson's
Corner, Virginia. Like many such centers in the United States, it
seems entirely strange and yet entirely familiar. Its strangeness
centers on the fact that it doesn't really seem to be located
anywhere: Tyson's Corner just looms up from the landscape
bordering the Leesburg Turnpike; a few miles down the road, it
just as abruptly winds down, its concentration of brick and glass
buildings, neon signs, and parking lots giving way to true country-

side where vegetables and horses and hay are still being raised. The familiarity of Tyson's Corner is that it contains a long row of stores, dominated by car dealers, whose large signs boast names better known to most Americans than their own genealogy: Woolco, Chevrolet, Fayva Shoes, Zayre, Cadillac, Toyota, Ford.

There are also the familiar deprivations of the American shopping center. Even a person willing to settle for some passable fast food, and not determined on anything as farfetched as nutrition, will find an attempt to eat at Tyson's Corner a frustrating occasion. How about a turkey sandwich on whole wheat with mayo? At a fast-food outlet in Tyson's Corner, this request will bring some "pressed" turkey that, like most meatish products pressed together from fat and leftovers, probably contains a high level of various additives, particularly the potentially very carcinogenic preservative nitrite. The pressed meat will be served on white bread "because we don't have any whole wheat" and slathered with imitation mayonnaise "because we don't have real mayonnaise." Yet just down the road, barely out of sight, silver-painted silos stand before the plowed fields and people are selling garden tomatoes and home-pressed apple cider from the roadside stands in front of their farms; their hand-lettered signs promise these products contain "no pesticides" and "no preservatives."

Right between these two representations of how people live—right where the commercial district winds down, and just before a farm offering "HAY BY THE BALE"—sits Hazleton Laboratories. Founded in 1946 by Dr. Lloyd Hazleton, Hazleton Laboratories is one of the first commercial testing labs in the country—a place where various companies send their new products and chemicals for an analysis of toxicity. Hazelton Laboratories was started in a toolshed and sits on property that was still farm when it got there. The first building seen along the driveway is actually an old red barn, now used for storage; behind lie the strict, sanitary, new cement-and-glass buildings where a large collection of rats, mice, guinea pigs, fruit flies, and other species live in scrubbed quarters watched over by human beings in white lab coats. It is the duty of these animals to react to new chemicals; it is the hope of the human beings that such reactions will suggest the possible health consequences of a substance in question for their own species.

Strapped between working farms and Tyson's Corner, Hazleton Laboratories could hardly have a more symbolic location. It is the price in experimental animals, fixating solutions, microscopes, chromosome analysis, sterile gloves, autopsies, and laboratory time that has to be paid to get to here from there—the price that, presumably, permits fresh farm products to be transposed into a pressed turkey sandwich on white with imitation mayo in safety. As many environmental debacles attest, however, the laboratory is not always as revealing as would be ideal. To the extent that the society has chosen Tyson's Corner over home-prepared apple cider, can it also predict and protect itself from drastic error?

In general, toxicity testing focuses, with varying degrees of success, on three main points: the mutagenicity, teratogenicity, and carcinogenicity of environmental agents. At present, the laboratory results from testing carcinogens are probably the most readily applied to human health. There are some two dozen agents, ranging from cigarette smoke to asbestos, that are well documented to cause cancer in humans. All of them—with the exception of arsenic—also cause cancer in various animals. It would seem that cancer initiation is a fairly standard response of living things to certain substances and that, in turn, evidence of cancer causation in animals is something humans should take seriously.

The great hindrances in cancer testing—as, indeed, in much of toxicity testing—are time and money. A typical test of one substance employs fifty or more animals, takes about two years, and costs some $200,000. To overcome both the statistical constraint of using so few animals and to compensate for the shorter life span of rodents, the animals are fed a much higher dose of the test substance than human beings might ordinarily encounter in their own environment; but, even at that rate, some observers estimate that "rigorous" animal experiments "could detect only those carcinogens which cause cancer at a rate greater than one out of 2,000 to 20,000 persons." There is, by the way, no truth in the widespread assumption that rats and mice are uniformly more susceptible to carcinogens than are primates just because they are smaller in size. Relative susceptibilities, instead, vary from chemical to chemical. With their faster rate of excreting PCBs, for example, rats can tolerate these widespread environmental contaminants at one hundred parts per million in their diet for well over a year without getting sick. Monkeys fed the same amount of PCBs for a year show "extreme morbidity and mortality," and tend to end up dead of several other causes even before they have time to respond to the carcinogenicity of PCBs by developing cancer.

The great quest in toxicity testing has been to discover so-called "rapid-assay" systems, which will bypass the months and money that animal testing consumes. The great breakthrough in this quest has been the Ames test, developed in the early 1970s by Dr. Bruce Ames, a professor of biochemistry at the University of California at Berkeley. Technically, since the Ames test involves seeing whether exposure to an agent will cause bacteria to mutate, it is a test of mutagenicity. However, since the evidence now suggests that "most, if not all, carcinogens are also mutagens," this device also serves to indicate carcinogenicity—and does so in a few days and for a few hundred dollars. Dr. Ames could have made an easy fortune from his test system, but did not choose to patent it; he said he did not see how he could be both making money from it and trying to encourage its use as an environmental protector at the same time. Even though no law yet actually requires the pretesting of new chemicals, many companies are now using the Ames test to analyze new products at an early stage of development and are abandoning carcinogenic ones before they are incorporated into consumer products.

As much of a breakthrough as it represents, however, the

Ames test—and the dozen or so other microbial rapid-assay systems since developed—does not signal that the day of dependable, rapid-assay testing is at hand. As time goes by, comparisons with their results and with the results of animal testing suggest that microbe-based systems might fail to detect about 30 percent of known carcinogens, among them organochlorine pesticides such as dieldrin and heptachlor, metals such as asbestos and hormones. Some of these problems may be overcome; others are probably insurmountable within the biological givens of microbial assays. Although the future will, without doubt, bring great improvements in rapid-assay assessments of carcinogenicity and mutagenicity, it is simply too early to abandon animal tests.

For the public, of course, carcinogenicity testing has formed one of the worst jolts of contemporary life. One favored or ubiquitous substance after another—saccharin, hair-dye ingredients, coal-tar food colors, asbestos, the flame retardant Tris—has been stamped malignant. There now seems to be a widespread public impression that any chemical, given to animals in large enough doses, will cause cancer; and along with this impression has come a general conclusion that technological societies can hardly function without substantially acceding to the use of carcinogens.

On the contrary, the general trend in carcinogenicity testing has been to suggest that technology and cancer hardly need walk hand in hand. In September 1978, Umberto Saffioti of the National Cancer Institute told a reporter for *Science* that about 3,500 chemicals had, by then, been adequately tested in animals, and only about 750 had proven to be carcinogens. Since this testing has largely concentrated on those chemicals that, from their structures, might well be suspected of causing trouble, the percentage of carcinogens among all chemicals is evidently much lower; a few years ago, the EPA estimated that perhaps only 1 percent of chemicals are "important" carcinogens. Considering the thousands of chemicals permitted into the marketplace without the least testing—there are probably now about 2 billion chemicals in total, some 63,000 of which are in common use—we are truly lucky that our retrospective discoveries of error have not been much worse.

Ferreting out any "important carcinogens" left among the mass of still-untested chemicals may not even require that great an investment of time or money. By "employing usage patterns as a criteria [for priority in testing]," Dr. Marvin Legator, a University of Texas geneticist, has pointed out, "what seems like an overwhelming task reduces to a reasonable number of chemicals. For example, 200 prescription drugs control 69 percent of the market; this translates into 190 separate ingredients. The non-prescription or over-the-counter (OTC) drug market contains as many as 500,000 products . . . [but] it is felt the number of active ingredients does not exceed 300. . . . Once again, as variegated and voluminous market as that of pesticides can be managed by concentrating on the market leaders: 19 fungicides, 37 herbicides, and 31 insecticides control 94 percent, 98 percent and 93 percent of their respective markets."

A good degree of safety, in short, would seem to be achieved by even minimal carcinogenicity testing—especially for the fetus. Something to keep in mind in discussions of the testing and regulation of carcinogens is the accumulating evidence that many such substances are fetotoxic in ways that range far beyond cancer. DES, for instance, also caused genital abnormalities; and cigarettes cause a considerable number of miscarriages. Controlling carcinogens might well result in avoiding much other injury to the unborn.

In contrast to carcinogen testing, with both its advances in rapid-assay systems and its close correlation in results between animal and man, testing for teratogens remains an unwieldy and uncertain business. On the one hand, more than six hundred agents have been shown to cause visible deformities in animals. Dozens of them, such as natural gas, the preservative EDTA, and aspirin, are in common use. Quite obviously, were even a fraction of these animal teratogens teratogenic to humans at amounts commonly encountered in the environment, few visibly normal children would be born. On the other hand, the differences in the biology of gestation are such that some agents that are relatively harmless to animals apparently are devastating to the human fetus. This, at least, was the case with thalidomide. After-the-fact research has revealed that the human fetus is sixty times more sensitive to thalidomide than unborn mice, one hundred times more sensitive than rats, two hundred times more than dogs, and seven hundred times more than the little hamster.

Teratogenicity testing itself remains a ponderous and time-consuming procedure. The routine at Hazleton Laboratories is quite standard. Ruth Durloo, the resident teratology researcher, first came to Hazleton in 1949 when the lab was still located in a farm shed. She wanted to work there, she notes rather ironically, because it was "way out in the country and a very relaxed place with plenty of fresh air around." Now, a lot of the fresh air is gone and the area near the lab has transformed itself entirely; but to try to determine whether a test chemical directly damages the fetus, Mrs. Durloo still employs techniques that have remained unchanged for years.

About sixty to ninety pregnant animals in total are exposed to each chemical being tested—usually at three different dose levels. "A few days before delivery," Mrs. Durloo goes on, "we remove the young by caesarean. With rats you usually get about twelve to fifteen pups and then they are divided, half to be examined viscerally and half to be examined skeletally." Those to be examined viscerally—or for aberrations of the internal organs— are put into a fixative known as Bouin's Solution, which "smells like the dickens" but which manages, after a week or so, both to render the soft tissues firm enough to cut and to soften the bones so they will yield to cutting. Mrs. Durloo then cross-sections them with a razor, rather like one would slice a small cucumber. By looking at the placement and shape of organs in these small cross-sections—from the positioning of the brain in the early slices to the shape of stomach and bowels revealed by later slices—Mrs. Durloo, with her practiced eye, can pick up small nuances in the development of the animals.

The fetuses to be examined for skeletal malformations have, in the interim, been fixed in alcohol for a week and then soaked in various solutions, which work the neat trick of staining their bones pink while leaving their tissues clear and colorless. The net result is an oddly charming view of little one-and-a-half inch-long pink skeletons still held in place by muscles and tissues that are virtually invisible. Mrs. Durloo examines all the bones on these tiny skeletons, from the thirteen little pairs of ribs to the small foot and tail bones, making sure they are complete in number and normal in shape.

People do this sort of testing because at least if there is animal damage it would alert to the possibility of human damage—and because there are very occasional correlations. For example, prenatally exposing male mice to DES produces virtually the same genital abnormalities seen in male humans exposed to DES. On the whole, however, teratogenicity testing as done today is a sort of desperation exercise—not unlike army foot maneuvers in a nuclear age. It is quite obvious that real breakthroughs are not going to come from this endless process of dosing mice and rats with possible teratogens and counting up their bones; the real breakthroughs depend on understanding the mechanisms and metabolism of teratogenesis.

Potentially, teratogens could work through any number of pathways, both in the mother and fetus. They could interfere with oxygen transfer from the mother, block the migration of embryonic cells, throw off the endocrine systems of both mother and fetus, or outrightly kill large numbers of fetal cells. In an example of the concentration on metabolism that may yet provide some basic answers about teratogenesis, two researchers at Johns Hopkins not long ago proposed a theory of oxygen transference, which they said might explain a slew of obstetric problems from the underweight babies often born to cigarette smokers to the increased malformation rate of the children of female operating-room personnel. This theory, which they developed after using a mass spectrometer to study the rates at which various gases cross sheep placenta, is that cytochrome P-450, an enzyme already well known to be the body's master drug metabolizer, may also be an important carrier of oxygen in the placenta. If, in fact, cytochrome P-450 does play a large role in the transfer of oxygen across the human placenta, the ingestion of the many drugs and substances known to bind to it—amphetamines, antihistamines, tranquilizers, the hydrocarbons in cigarette smoke—would interfere with its oxygen-binding capacity and slash the fetal oxygen supply. While this particular theory remains in the controversy stage, the basic focus on the pathways and metabolism of gestation is a crucial one.

Since the present testing of teratogens is so unreliable, human epidemiology again comes to the fore. Although epidemiology, in the past, has not proven very helpful in detecting teratogens already in the marketplace, it could, in the future, prove extremely helpful in catching any new teratogens—or major mutagens—before they wreaked their damage on very many children. This preventive approach has focused on the idea of monitoring spontaneously aborted fetuses for malformations or chromosome damage which might suggest that a dangerous substance had entered the human realm.

At the moment, a small group at the College of Physicians and Surgeons at Columbia University seems to be the only one in the world engaged in constant monitoring of spontaneous abortions. Started in 1974 and headed by Zena Stein, a professor of epidemiology at Columbia, this group—which does not even have a formal name—examines all the fetuses expelled during sponta-neous abortions at three major New York hospitals. They try to determine whether each aborted fetus is abnormal in appearance or chromosome structure and whether the mother had any unusual environmental exposure that might account for the mis-carriage; they also gather ongoing information about factors ranging from the parents' employment to the mother's use of coffee and vaginal deodorants, which they are analyzing for any steady links with miscarriage.

As an adjunct to the furor over abortion, there is also a growing furor over "fetal research." It is hard to see, however, that there is a difference between, say, autopsying a dead adult and examining a few cells from a spontaneously aborted fetus. "A spontaneous abortus is an experiment which will never become human," Dr. Stein maintains, "so the least we can do is try to use it to protect humans. If something really terrible does happen, this will be the first place we can find out."

The value of miscarriage monitoring was dramatically highlighted in late 1976 when, at one of the hospitals the Stein group monitors, there was a four-fold increase in the number of spontaneously aborted fetuses with Down's syndrome. This increase tapered down after a few months; but it left behind several questions. Why only one hospital? Why had it ended? Was it a chance occurrence or a real increase?

Some months later, the Stein group learned that a consumer product, which was rather quickly withdrawn because of its toxicity on other counts, had been briefly test-marketed in the area of New York served by the one hospital. They also found out that, in 1977, an unusual number of babies with even more severe chromosome defects had been born in a city where the test product was manufactured; these babies were conceived during precisely the same months as the Down's fetuses in New York were conceived. It was, however, too late to trace all the Down's mothers and inquire whether they had used the test product. The clue may be nothing more than coincidence. The Stein group is, however, convinced of one thing—that this Down's outbreak was too large to be caused by chance. It had a decided, if still unknown, cause.

Obviously, had the four-fold increase in spontaneously aborted Down's fetuses continued, there would have been a massive epidemiological hunt for the cause; and by beginning it six months before an increase in actual Down's births showed itself, everyone would have been that much further ahead in halting the continued exposure of other mothers to the guilty agent. This program of spontaneous abortion monitoring costs about $300,000 a year. Considering that the lifetime costs of institutionalizing one child with severe Down's syndrome or other serious damage are now reaching toward a million dollars, the program would pay for three years of operations simply by discovering a serious mutagen or teratogen in time to prevent injury to one extra baby. It may well be a sign of the universe's benign intentions toward us that so fundamentally careless a society—a society that declines to accord the proper respect to even that animal evidence that is available—can obtain this fundamental protection for so small an expenditure.

It is perhaps natural that research should concentrate on the obvious physical events of cancer, mutation, and birth defects. As more has been learned about subtler damage to humans, however, it has come to seem that this, too, deserves more research attention. Dr. Robert Miller's views on the subject are of interest. Contrary to what might be presumed of someone who is head of the clinical epidemiology branch of the National Cancer Institute and past chairman of the Environmental Hazards Committee of the American Academy of Pediatrics, neither cancer nor visible birth defects are the environmental disorders that chiefly concern him. The first item on Dr. Miller's list of concerns is damage to the immature brain—a subject, he points out, about which we know very little, by comparison with the present understanding of cancer.

There are various reasons that he, and some other observers, name this priority. In the first place, the prospects for curing cancer certainly seem brighter than the prospects of learning to replace damaged or fully destroyed brain cells. Although few cancer specialists think that the "magic bullet" for cancer is right around the corner, recent years have brought great strides in arresting some forms of the disease, prominent among them juvenile leukemia. By contrast, no one has ever reconstructed the brain of a mercury- or lead-poisoned child, and this seems a feat that will long—perhaps always—remain beyond the reach of medicine.

In the second place, as serious a disease as cancer is, at least it does not usually strike until middle age or later; the great period for vulnerability to brain damage seems to extend from the fetal period to about age two and a half or three. During that period, very small amounts of some chemicals seem able to exact damage that will only get worse with time and that as effectively forbid a child to take part in society as some forms of physical crippling; many lead-damaged children, for example, may experience great difficulty learning in school despite having quite normal intelligence.

This is not to say cancer should not be a focus of worry; it *is* worrisome, and the situation is only likely to get worse as past years of carelessness with carcinogens take their toll. Aside from concerns about human suffering, it seems a blunt question whether the industrial societies can even afford the amount of cancer cases they seem destined to accumulate. With a fatal cancer case often costing $20,000, and with cures or "remissions" sometimes involving one, two, or more years of intensive chemotherapy, cancer would seem to loom as much as a cause of national bankruptcy as of mortality.

Still, Dr. Miller wonders whether the medical and public preoccupation with cancer—or at least some common ways of expressing this preoccupation—hasn't become "a public health hazard in itself." It troubles him, for example, to see so much research money poured into the sort of environmental studies that consume a few million dollars to show there are a few extra cancer cases among the workers in some particular industry. Although a believer in the many uses of epidemiology, he thinks this sort of money might better be applied to basic research. "You never know where the breaks are going to come from," he comments, citing the example of the Ames test—which came into existence not because Dr. Ames was looking for a rapid-assay carcinogen test, but because he had spent many years studying the genes of bacteria.

It also troubles Dr. Miller—and, certainly, other people—that cancer has to a large extent become the sole criterion for judging environmental quality and the need to ban various substances. A few years ago, at a conference on water pollution sponsored by the New York Academy of Sciences, the participants typically spent a good deal of time trying to correlate various pollutants in local water supplies with the cancer rates of nearby communities; yet water pollution episodes in both the United States and other nations have done a good deal more than possibly cause cancer. "It is clear," Dr. Miller remarked, "that the contamination of water has shrunk the size of newborn babies, starved others for oxygen, pustulated the skin for years in persons of all ages, caused bones to ache with every step, and addled the brains of newborns, children, and adults. With this array of adverse effects on the integrity of the human organism, is there really any need to invoke the specter of cancer to achieve clean water?"

The story of cyclamates provides perhaps as graphic an example as there is that early brain damage may be as much a hazard as cancer. This banned artificial sweetener is recognizably among the mildest of carcinogens; it is actually less threatening than the saccharin that is now, in turn, a focus of controversy. As weak a carcinogen as it may be, however, preliminary testing of cyclamates—testing abandoned after its disgrace—suggested that it perhaps had no small impact on the developing brain. In 1969, David Stone, who was then Senior Scientist at the Worcester (Mass.) Foundation for Experimental Biology, fed pregnant rats relatively low levels of cyclamates and found that their offspring were both hyperactive in behavior and slow to learn to respond to a food reward. Dr. Stone was moved by these animal observations to question several hundred mothers of both retarded and normally intelligent children about their eating habits. It turned out that significantly more mothers of retarded children than of normal ones had consumed artificial sweeteners while pregnant.

This outcome does not necessarily mean that artificial sweeteners cause mental retardation. It could be that intelligent women—who may in any case be destined to have more intelligent children—eat more soundly; it could be that some of the many other suspect additives that tend to be used in artificially sweetened sodas and food were the culprits. In view, however, of the jumpy behavior of rats prenatally exposed to cyclamates, a difference in behavior among the normally intelligent children, which seemed to coordinate with their mothers' consumption of artificial sweeteners, may be quite telling. Some 4.3 percent of the mothers who used these sweeteners while pregnant described their normally intelligent children as being hyperactive, or very nervous, or very irritable—a description that fewer than 1 percent of the non-sweetener-using mothers applied to their normal children. At the least, these combined observations suggest it would be as useful to have a means of predicting fetal brain injury as to have a reliable rapid-assay test for chemical carcinogenicity.

At present, then, protecting the species from environmental harm remains a fairly plodding matter of doing animal studies and backing them with human epidemiology. Obviously the goal is to come to reliable conclusions about the risks and benefits of various chemicals, products, and medical procedures. But the data yielded by such efforts are often open to a wide range of interpretation. Some people think that the reason young men are dying from heart attacks in North Karelia, Finland, is that their diet is loaded with cheese, butter, and other fatty foods; others think they may be at least partially victim to a radar facility. Some observers judge the mutagenic danger of X rays from the Hiroshima bomb survivors, whose children do not seem to have "significant" genetic damage; others judge X-ray dangers from several studies that suggest that three or four abdominal X rays would about double a woman's chance of having a child with Down's Syndrome. To some observers, 2,4,5-T is a cause of birth defects in Vietnam and miscarriages in Oregon; to Dow Chemical, it has not yet been proved that "properly applied" 2,4,5-T has harmed a single human being on the face of this earth. To Thomas Corbett, the young anesthesiologist who has done much work on the toxicity of anesthesia, it "would require an extraordinarily recalcitrant bias not to consider the chronic exposure to low concentrations of anesthetic gases to be responsible for the excess incidence of cancer and birth defects seen among operating room personnel." By contrast, Dr. Louis Ferstandig, a chemist who is Technical Director of Halocarbon Laboratories, a New Jersey anesthesia manufacturer, recently announced in *Anesthesia and Analgesia,* the journal of the International Anesthesia Research Society, that "there are no statistically sound studies which prove that trace concentrations of anesthetic gases exert harmful effects."

Although it may sometimes seem that these differences in interpretation largely depend on whether the interpreter is speaking for industry or in some public interest role, sometimes opinions on evidence are so divergent that whole nations end up individually immersed in tragedies that other countries manage to avoid. The thalidomide tragedy, for example, was largely a European one. The United States has only a handful of thalidomide children, whose mothers were given the drug on an experimental basis. Dr. Frances Kelsey, then a Food and Drug Administration medical officer, long delayed the general use of thalidomide in the United States by demanding basic toxicity tests which no European country had previously thought to demand. More than that, two American drug companies also contributed to the American escape from thalidomide. The German manufacturer of the drug had first sought out Smith Kline & French to be its American licensee. After testing thalidomide on animals for two years, Smith Kline & French turned it down, as later did Lederle Laboratories— not because they had stumbled across evidence of its fetal effects, but because they could find no evidence it functioned particularly well as a tranquilizer. Yet, in Europe, thalidomide was not only then one of the most profitable and largest-selling drugs, but was also widely regarded as an almost magic tranquilizer, representing a real breakthrough for that type of drug.

By contrast—perhaps just because they had the inescapable lesson of their mangled thalidomide babies always before them— European countries largely avoided the DES tragedy. In the United States, at least several hundred thousand and possibly a few million pregnant women were prescribed this drug; in

England, fewer than 10,000 were. The hard, practical, wary Israelis, rather surprisingly, may have been the only people who used relatively more hormone supports during pregnancy than did Americans.

These are major lessons for Westerners to keep in mind through all their self-concepts of their "rationality," "objectivity," and "scientific thinking." Nonetheless, even in error and confusion, decisions have to be made. Are new products too risky? Should old chemicals now under suspicion be banned? Where much is implied and less is conclusive, the protection of the public does not just depend on studies' being done; it also depends on their reasoned and reasonable interpretation.

The value of the evidence for or against a substance in question largely depends on three points: the design, or "protocol," of the studies, their statistical "significance," and their cumulative impact. One study is virtually never enough—whether done on humans or in animals—and it is all the better when effects can be shown in at least two, if not more, species. Obviously, it is a good deal easier to control the design of animal studies than of human studies. In the laboratory, both the animals being tested and the control animals against which they are compared can be kept in strictly the same environment and given strictly the same food, water, and handling. No matter how well done an animal study, however, there is always the nagging matter of its true meaning for humans.

The major disadvantage of human epidemiology is that the human environment is simply "uncontrollable." Some of the studies showing high rates of birth defects in some industrial areas have, for example, stalled on blazing arguments over the matter of local wind conditions: in other words, would the wind actually have blown the presumably guilty factory emissions toward those homes where there was a malformed child in the family?

The interpretation of birth-defect studies is particularly hard because picking up minor malformations, and even some major ones, requires a practiced eye. For all that the children of alcoholic women are now said to have a rather high incidence of major malformations, they really do not look that different from other children—which, no doubt, accounts for the centuries of failure to detect their problem. Their craniofacial abnormalities, particularly their somewhat flattened "pug" noses, tend to give them, if anything, a rather appealing, childish demeanor. The real importance of their outward "malformations" lies in their so often being the sign of a wrecked brain.

Although there are accepted international standards for the diagnosis of birth defects, clearly no one will ever control what doctors, researchers, and other fallible humans manage to see. Virtually every effort—and there have been many—to sit down and "really decide" the rate of birth defects has stumbled into inconclusiveness. Several years ago, for example, research groups in both Madison, Wisconsin, and Albany, New York, determined to count up all the subtle defects—down to such things as slightly askew palm creases—to be found among a group of newborns. The Madison group counted up a rate of subtle defects among its newborns of 14.1 percent: the Albany group counted a rate of 33 percent. Meanwhile, although newborns in the Collaborative Perinatal population were intensely studied, the Project did not, at the time, manage to act as an alert to the substantial increase in severe malformations caused by the 1964 rubella (German measles) epidemic. The perception of birth defects, in short, can range from the extreme of overlooking major teratogens such as alcohol and thalidomide to the extreme of pronouncing virtually everyone to be malformed—precise placement of every last nuance, from earlobes to toenails, not being the fate of very many people.

Aside from a design that at least manages to control for obvious variables, from the scientific point of view, the next important measure of whether data mean anything is that the results be "statistically significant." For the most part, data are considered statistically significant when various mathematical tests and calculations show that the alleged effect would not happen by chance more than 5 percent of the time—although researchers may also sometimes use both tighter and looser criteria of significance. The great argument sometimes directed at this methodology is that *statistical* significance may not always be a measure of *social* significance. The widespread use of drugs or chemicals with side effects too rare to show up in an epidemiological study as statistically significant may nonetheless pose no small cumulative problem.

A very important dispute over what is statistically and socially significant has, for example, focused on the question of whether women who conceive within the first few months—but especially within the first month—of halting birth control pills are slightly more likely to have malformed children; obviously, with oral contraceptives being used by about sixty million women worldwide, even a slight risk of this sort would result in literally thousands of malformed children.

The question first arose with several studies in the late 1960s and early 1970s, which showed that conceptuses spontaneously aborted from women who conceived within three months or so of halting oral contraceptive use had an unusual rate of both severe chromosome defects and physical abnormalities. Since the damage seemed so severe that any embryo with these injuries was almost bound to abort early in gestation, no one was particularly worried about these findings. Moreover, a few other studies did not detect severe damage in the aborted embryos of former pill users. As time went by, however, researchers began to consider that there should be more careful study of post-pill children.

In 1974, for example, Dr. Dwight Janerich, then director of the New York State Birth Defects Institute, was comparing various hormone exposures among some one hundred children with limb-reduction deformities and one hundred normal children when he learned that six of the malformed children in his study group had been conceived within three months of their mothers' having halted oral contraceptive use; only one of the normal children had been conceived within that time period.

As it happens, the Russians had years earlier made oblique reference to limb reduction deformities among children born to their own pill users. In 1967, then–Soviet Health Minister Boris Petrovski, in a rare interview, told a group of American journalists that the Soviet Union had decided against general use of oral contraceptives "because we do not want our children being born with deformed hands and feet." While it seems more likely that the constant Russian worry about being underpopulated accounts as much as anything for their ban on oral contraceptives, it is certainly striking that the Russians confronted the possibility of birth defects much sooner than did Western researchers.

Larger, more detailed studies that focused on conceptions in the first few months after halting pill use have not settled this question. *The Pill and Births: The Jerusalem Study*, published in 1978, is the largest study to date of post-pill births and reports on the pregnancies of almost 16,000 non-pill users and former pill users. In recently resifting the data from this study, Dr. Susan Harlap, the chief researcher, found "no excess of major congenital malformations in the children of women who conceived within the first month of halting pills." As, however, she noted in the introduction to *The Pill and Births*, three other large, prospective studies of post-pill children (two of these studies are English and one is French) "did show overall excesses of malformations in the pill group," although these were not statistically significant.

The largest American study to date of post-pill births was published in late 1978 and also seemed to hint at some trouble. In a survey of almost 7,000 pregnancies, Dr. Kenneth J. Rothman of the Harvard School of Public Health found that when the mother conceived within a month of stopping pill use, the children had a malformation rate of 4.3 percent; when the mother had never used pills or had stopped them for at least three years before conceiving, the malformation rate was 3.3 percent. To Dr. Rothman, "a reasonable interpretation of these data would be that oral contraceptives present no major teratogenic hazards"—an interpretation that brought an angry rebuttal from Dr. Irwin Bross, the chief biostatistician at Roswell Park Memorial Institute, a major research center in Buffalo, New York. This conclusion, Dr. Bross countered in the *New England Journal of Medicine,* was "a basic mistake." He pointed out that, even though the results were not "statistically significant," there was still about a one-third higher rate of malformation among children conceived in the first month after pills were halted.

At this point, more evidence pointed toward some occasional problems in the first few months after stopping pills than toward this period's being entirely safe for conception. Oral contraceptives, on the other hand, are hardly in the same category of risk evaluation as plastic seat covers, spray cans, "non-dairy" creamers, and some of the other flotsam and jetsam of sleazy technology. Oral contraceptives are intended to fulfill a real human need. Their very occasional lethal effects to women themselves are relatively minor compared with the chances of dying during pregnancy and childbirth throughout much of the globe; and if they do occasionally cause birth defects, by providing reliable contraception for older women they have also prevented the births of massive numbers of malformed children.

Dealing with this possible risk does not, however, require dumping all oral contraceptives into the ocean; it simply requires informing pill users to be careful. Dr. Janerich, for one, thinks that oral contraceptives "may possibly be the most important medical advance of this century." He also thinks that "if there is a safer way to use them, people should be told about it."

Since April 1977, the Food and Drug Administration has required that the patient inserts for oral contraceptives contain the brief advice to "wait a few months after stopping the pill before you try to become pregnant. During those few months, use another form of contraception." Whether these two small-print sentences actually constitute giving women fair warning about a simple action that might guard their children from as much as a one-third increase in risk of malformation is debatable. As of 1976, 22.5 percent of the married women in the United States between the ages of fifteen and forty-five were using oral contraceptives. The government sponsors public education campaigns on plenty of other subjects. It would not be unreasonable for some government agency to occasionally include a message about the proper use of oral contraceptives among the late-night television messages concerning the purchase of payroll savings bonds, seatbelt safety in automobiles, and the avoidance of forest fires.

Dr. Harlap, meanwhile, while basically concluding that "fears of possible effects on future pregnancies need not deter [the vast majority of women] from choosing oral contraceptives," finds it appalling that, in the post-thalidomide age, pills were used for almost fifteen years before there was an appropriately large-scale effort to determine possible adverse effects on reproduction and the fetus. What drug, after all, could have been more deserving of scrutiny for possible reproductive effects from the beginning of its use than a drug specifically targeted to interfere with the normal function of the reproductive system? There is an old street saying that advises "If you can't do the time, don't do the crime." Like other similarly belated questions, the belated questions about the pill suggest that, in the world as it runs today, similar advice might be "If you can't do the epidemiology, don't use the technology."

In recent years, much attention has focused on amniocentesis and other techniques of prenatal diagnosis. During amniocentesis, a needle is used to withdraw from the uterus about 20 milliliters of the amniotic fluid cushioning the fetus. By analyzing fetal cells that have sloughed off into the fluid, physicians can now detect some one hundred genetic diseases—including Down's syndrome. Components of the fluid itself can also to some extent reveal whether the fetus has a neural tube defect; and, with techniques of prenatal blood monitoring now being refined, the early diagnosis of some blood disorders, such as sickle cell anemia and Cooley's anemia, has become possible.

Amniocentesis is usually performed in the fourth month of

pregnancy. Obviously, the main reason for early diagnosis is that the parents can choose to abort an abnormal fetus. The association with abortion has made the technique controversial. It seems only fair to point out that the technique has more often been responsible for people's having children than it has been a prelude to abortion. Before the reassurance of prenatal diagnosis became widely available, people who knew they had a history of serious genetic disease in their families, or who had already given birth to a seriously diseased child, simply did not dare to initiate pregnancies.

Some of the present attitudes toward amniocentesis, however, seem misguided—not to say occasionally rather disturbing. There is great medical enthusiasm for amniocentesis, and stories in the general press have talked rather breathlessly about the possibility it presents of "wiping out genetic disease" (something which, by the way, will not be wiped out as long as there are genes) and of "making more perfect babies" (whatever a "more perfect" baby may be). Although people do not publicly discuss amniocentesis in terms of an environmental "solution," it is hard not to detect an unstated note to this enthusiasm—a lurking idea that amniocentesis may substantially "solve" the problem of birth defects, whether environmentally or naturally caused, simply by eliminating the defective fetuses. If there is no conscious advocacy to depend on amniocentesis in this way, there may well be a subconscious flagging in the tedious research and care required to prevent environmental damage to the unborn in the first place.

Perhaps in a country where induced abortion has essentially been accepted as a civil right, to make various moral distinctions about the uses of abortion is irrelevant. But to depend on prenatal diagnosis to deal with environmental harm to the fetus reaches far beyond abortion: it would place women in the wrenching position of being experimental breeders; it would require that they sit by for four months or longer to see whether they had managed, through the chemical carelessness around them, to conceive a normal child; it is insupportable. And, more than that, any idea that prenatal diagnosis will substantially save us from environmental errors could be a grave delusion.

At present, amniocentesis is basically limited to determining genetic defects. Except, perhaps, for the limited case of neural tube defects, it does not reveal direct teratogenic injury to the fetus; and while sonar does now offer the possibility of detecting some types of physical malformations fairly early in gestation, it is still hard to see that there could ever be prenatal detection of some of the injuries it might be most useful to understand—including some types of retardation, blindness, and deafness—or those few cells somewhere in the fetus that have been transformed by a transplacental carcinogen and are destined to turn rampantly malignant some years later. Prenatal detection would simply not have "eliminated" some of the worst current environmental calamities. It could not have spotted the DES children or those multitudes of children in the Minamata area who are "mentally deficient" despite having escaped actual physical malformation from mercury.

Even in the realm of genetic disorders, amniocentesis is largely limited to the detection of syndromes and crippling caused by fairly obvious chromosome disorders. Detecting the "smaller" mutations, which may, in their fashion, be just as crucial to function, awaits the detailed unraveling of the genetic code—an event presumably many years, not to say decades, in the future. Lowering the rate of some types of obvious malformation through the use of amniocentesis might well engender a very false sense of security. It is not going to do much good to have all these "more perfect"-looking babies—babies who don't have Down's syndrome and who don't have spina bifida—should some large portion of them not be able to read and write, be destined to develop cancer when they are sixteen, break down fairly early in life like Spyker's mice, or sustain so many "minor" mutations that they fulfill Herman Muller's vision of a future where people are "devoted chiefly to the effort to live carefully, to spare and prop up their own feebleness . . ."

Amniocentesis, in short, may be a helpful and reassuring procedure for some individuals; but it hardly offers a general escape from environmental responsibility. If there are "magic" solutions to human reproduction and the problems of protecting the fetus, they lie in such directions as genetic engineering and growing fetuses in test tubes—where they would be wrapped in protective devices rather like those straws that come in white wrappers bearing the legend "Sanitized for Your Own Protection." At that point, the human race may communally decide they are Luddites at heart and say no.

Amniocentesis, moreover, evidently has its own hazards, which, if rare, certainly require further analysis. The most detailed study of children born after amniocentesis is a report of the Medical Research Council Working Party on Amniocentesis—an English group—which was published in late 1978 as a supplement to the *British Journal of Obstetrics and Gynecology.* The Medical Research Council group found that children whose mothers had had amniocentesis seemed to have from 1 to 1.5 percent more major orthopedic postural abnormalities and unexplained respiratory difficulties at birth than did a control group of children whose mothers had not had amniocentesis.

The Medical Research Council group also felt that the excess risk of spontaneous abortion following amniocentesis was at least 1 percent and that another 1 percent of babies had died at around the time of birth from various obstetric complications—hemorrhage requiring emergency caesarean deliveries, placental complications—also quite probably attributable to the procedure. Doctors at the Prenatal Detection Program of the University of California at San Francisco have also recently said they are "reasonably certain" that some small number of spontaneous abortions, although probably fewer than found in the Medical Research Council study, occur in the wake of amniocentesis.

These are not devastating findings—on the whole, for example, after monitoring 3,000 procedures, the University of Southern California physicians concluded that prenatal diagnosis was "safe, highly reliable, and extremely accurate"—but any amount of hazard does take amniocentesis out of the realm of the routine. In trying to balance its apparent hazards against the potential of detecting an abnormal fetus, the Medical Research Council report suggested that some indications seemed more justified than others. When, for example, the parents had previously had children with certain abnormalities, the chance of detecting another abnormal fetus was quite high. By contrast, the Medical Research Council group did not think that maternal age really became a justifiable criterion for amniocentesis until the mother reached age forty. In the thirty-five-to-thirty-nine-year-old group—thirty-five is now often the recommended age for beginning amniocentesis—only 0.8 percent of women were carrying a Down's fetus; this increased to 4.1 percent between the ages of forty and forty-one, 6.5 percent between forty-two and forty-three, and 14.6 percent between forty-four and forty-seven.

The Medical Research Council observations are not, of course, final; they are simply part of the ongoing work needed to quantify the risks and benefits of what is a fairly new procedure. Another caution is that all the follow-up of post-amniocentesis children to date has consisted of monitoring them immediately after birth or, at most, at age one. Amniocentesis may or may not involve longer-term hazards, particularly from the use of sonar and local anesthesia, which usually accompany the procedure. In the Collaborative Perinatal population, for example, when the mother had been given a shot of novocain—a local anesthetic quite commonly administered before amniocentesis—during pregnancy, the child's risk of developing a central nervous system malignancy before age eight increased ninefold. Although this observation diminishes somewhat in intensity from being based on very few cancer cases, it does clearly invite further study.

Some physicians and technicians use sonar to guide the needle during the procedure and others use it to check on the internal situation before they proceed. In either case, an exposure to ultrasound is now common during amniocentesis procedures in this country. While sonar is, without doubt, a wonderful invention and a superior diagnostic tool, it is not free of all hazard. Exposing unborn animals to diagnostic intensities of this acoustic energy has provoked an array of biological effects, including delayed neuromuscular development in fetal rats, brain damage and immunoglobic depression in mice, and EEG aberrations in young monkeys.

There has been enough follow-up of human children exposed to ultrasound in early pregnancy to provide substantial reassurance that it does not cause them severe malformations. There is, however, some fleeting evidence that infants exposed to ultrasound are slightly predisposed to develop infections, hearing deficits, and some small neurological quirks. The Bureau of Radiological Health is now engaged in an intensive five-year follow-up that involves comparing children exposed to ultrasound during amniocentesis to children whose aminocentesis did not include ultrasound. "All we are saying," sighs Dr. Charlotte Silverman, Deputy Director of the Division of Biological Effects of the Bureau of Radiological Health, "is that remembering some of the past problems we've had, for once let's do the follow-up first before everyone is exposed to the technology."

As amniocentesis becomes a more and more widely used procedure, even a possible 1 percent of postural abnormalities or a slight excess of hearing deficits would accumulate disturbingly. In England, at this point, while supporting the concept of amniocentesis, the Royal College of Obstetricians and Gynecologists has denounced as premature various government proposals to launch national programs for prenatal testing for certain disorders. In the United States, it seems that the place of this form of prenatal diagnosis in obstetric practice may essentially be decided—as more and more American medical practice in general is being decided—in the courts and by malpractice litigation. In late 1978, the New York Court of Appeals ruled that, in certain instances, doctors could be held liable for the lifetime special care of a deformed or defective child born when they failed to adequately advise the parents about the availability of genetic counseling and amniocentesis. Although no physician has in fact yet had to pay such a penalty, that it looms over them in theory may well mean that obstetricians will point their patients toward amniocentesis with considerable fervor.

*

When the question of banning chemicals or products is raised, there is often a lot of talk about the "scientific method" of evaluating the evidence. The scientific method essentially refers to testing things from every conceivable angle until the evidence for or against them can hardly be doubted. It means beginning with several animal tests in different species—tests that, preferably, show a dose-effect response. It means then proceeding to look for a human response, usually first through small, retrospective, case-control studies, and then through massive prospective studies. The difference between the two epidemiological methods is that one is random and one is not. In retrospective case-control studies, researchers look at a relatively small number of people already known to have a disease or disorder and try to determine whether more of them have been exposed to a suspect agent than a similar group of healthy people; it is a powerful, fairly quick tool for detecting human responses, but a tool that can just as quickly lead to error. A case-control study, for example, provided the swift, shattering kick that condemned DES as a carcinogen; but case-control studies have also put into circulation such mistaken notions as that hepatitis during pregnancy causes Down's syndrome, and that women who once took birth control pills have fewer than average male children.

Prospective studies, by contrast, involve following large populations fairly randomly exposed to environmental agents and watching for effects on their future health; they are often prohibitively expensive and time-consuming. The *Lancet* once pointed out that to prospectively "incriminate a substance which doubled the incidence of a birth defect with a normal incidence of 1 in 1,000, it would be necessary to study 23,000 newborns whose mothers had taken the substance." The Perinatal Collaborative Project is, of course, one of the major prospective efforts ever undertaken; the doctors, mothers, and babies involved in it just went about their normal business and researchers later attempted to determine whether the children's health was affected by factors ranging from their anesthesia exposure during birth to their parents' occupations. The Collaborative Perinatal Project is conservatively estimated to have cost $100 million so far—and all the information available has hardly yet been gleaned from the computer tapes. Merely analyzing the material on drugs and physical malformations that was contained in *Birth Defects and Drugs in Pregnancy* took six years, and ended up with the main participants' locking themselves in a house on Martha's Vineyard until they finished. By that time, they agreed on only two things—that they would never again undertake so massive a project and that they could hardly stand to look at one another for a single day more.

Industry will complain bitterly when its products are condemned without full benefit of the "scientific method." It is obvious, however, that there are not resources on the face of the earth to treat all suspect chemicals to this full inquiry. (It is also obvious that the true scientific method would have been to test these things properly in animals in the first place and closely watching for any human effects from their first entrance into the ecosystem.) What, then, should the guiding standard be? Dr. Howard Ulfelder has suggested one. "We can't be all science or all outrage," he suggests, "but in policing the environment enlightened humanitarianism should prevail over strictly scientific, statistical demands for proofs."

Dr. Ulfelder is in a position to comment. When head of the Department of Gynecology at Massachusetts General Hospital, he was the first person to suspect that DES had caused genital cancers in human females; although much of his data for this suspicion came from his own observations—a source that researchers are naturally prejudiced toward accepting—he still could hardly believe it; DES and cancer, however, is one connection that has proved conclusive.

Men are naturally most impressed by
diseases which have obvious manifestations. Yet some of their worst enemies
creep on them unobtrusively.

DR. RENÉ DUBOS
*Mirage of Health*

# Chapter 4

# NERVOUS NERVES

Among the mysteries of childhood is a disorder known as hyperkinesis or hyperactivity, which snatches away normal behavioral control from its young victims. They break into frantic
motion—motion that ranges from the merely annoying to the
dangerous. They live in a bizarre world where their conscious
minds struggle toward normalcy, but their bodies seem to have
assumed an angry, restless life of their own. Hyperactive children
lash out wildly at themselves and others; they will assault siblings,
set fires, or compulsively bang their own heads against a wall.
In a diary account of just ten minutes from "an ordinary day"

in the life of her nine-year-old hyperactive son, a Tennessee mother describes the child's attempt to do homework. It comes at the close of an afternoon already marked by the boy's having set two fires, kicked a woman neighbor, and smashed his few remaining toys to bits. "Child bangs door, slumps in chair, snaps point of pencil, jumps on furniture, scratches paper, plays with toes, knocks over lamp, constant wiggles, loud noises," reads the entry. "Mother gives up."

Once considered a rare disorder, hyperactivity has, within the past decade, become what is sometimes said to be the fastest-growing childhood affliction in the United States. There are some identifiable causes of hyperactivity, including brain damage at birth, hypoglycemia, and psychological trauma, but millions of dollars in research effort have failed to identify a generally accepted cause for the majority of cases. And, in the absence of a cure, medicine has adopted the common if dubious practice of controlling these children with drugs. The products used to medicate them are often derived from amphetamines, the same drugs known in the vernacular as "speed." These "pediatric" amphetamines do not "cure" the basic disorder. They act, instead, as a sort of pharmaceutical straitjacket to keep children still—so still that some school systems now have cots for drugged pupils who habitually fall asleep. Current sales figures suggest that not fewer than 500,000, and probably closer to one million American children, the bulk under ten years of age, are now tethered to psychotropic, or behavior-altering, medication.

There is, however, an exception to this medical stalemate. American medicine has been truly distinguished by a hard core of brilliant clinical allergists who have been at the forefront of environmental interest and who have looked to diet, allergy, and sensitivities as important causes of youthful malaise, whether behavioral or physical. Around 1958, long before many "coal-tar" colors were recognized as being carcinogenic to animals, alert allergists were already reporting that these dyes could cause asthma attacks in susceptible youngsters. And, as long ago as 1947, Dr. Theron C. Randolph of Chicago was writing in the *Journal of*

*Pediatrics* of children driven almost loony by allergic reactions. Randolph launched his observations on behavior and allergy with natural causes of allergy; but he has come to consider synthetic chemicals and pollutants as the real allergic banes of society.

To an amazing extent, the rest of the medical profession regarded these early insights from the environmental battleground as a rumor of war in a distant province. Not until the early 1970s did the war really come home. It was then that Dr. Benjamin F. Feingold, a California allergist in his early seventies, began announcing—not in medical journals, but on television and in a best-selling book—that about half of hyperactive children would return to normal or near-normal behavior when put on a diet free of synthetic colors and flavors. Painfully, the realization that the immature nervous system is a prime target of environmental toxins began to work its way into general awareness. It is curious that many people, physicians included, are readier to accept the idea that some synthetic additives may cause cancer—which, after all, is a major biological event—than that some substances may handicap the nervous system, a part of the body in especially delicate balance. But Dr. Feingold, who had not become concerned about the question of environment and behavior until very late in life, was the first to recognize the difficulty. "People think you're a little nuts when you first tell them a food additive can make a child violent," he observes with a congenial smile. "It takes a while to sink in."

When Dr. Feingold retired in the early 1970s as the chief of allergy at the Kaiser-Permenente Medical Center in San Francisco, he had spent fifty years in medicine, the first half as a pediatrician and the second as an allergist. A succession of incidents during this long, combined career had finally convinced him that some food additives, predominantly the colors and flavors, can trigger the bizarre behavior symptomatic of hyperkinesis. The first clue had actually surfaced in the unexpected shape of a forty-year-old woman who appeared at Kaiser-Permenente suffering from what he retrospectively refers to as "a very fortunate case of giant hives." Feingold advised her to eliminate two groups of substances from her diet. The first included synthetic colors and flavors, and the second, all foods and medicines containing the salicylate radical. (The salicylate radical is a certain group of atoms found in aspirin, tea, one vegetable—cucumbers—and several fruits, among them apples, tomatoes, oranges, and peaches.) For reasons not entirely understood, the salicylate radical and the synthetic colors and flavors all can act as culprits in the outbreak of hives and other rashes. Banning them has become a routine procedure.

At the time, however, a ban on all three together was rather a new tactic. It quickly conquered the hives, but it also brought Feingold an excited call from the chief of psychiatry at Kaiser, who briskly inquired what the allergy department had "done to that woman?" It seemed that soon after her hives subsided, so had the angry, hostile behavior for which she was in therapy. Feingold dismissed this first suggestion of a link between food additives and behavior as coincidence, and some years passed before the continuing reports of behavior changes associated with the elimination diet finally inspired him to investigate a specific link to hyperkinesis. There was logic in the thought that substances that seemed to unhinge an occasional adult might have an especially savage effect on the young.

Using his retirement to translate his suspicions into a treatment program, he first launched four hyperactive children on a diet that, modeled after the one prescribed for the "fortunate case of hives," banned salicylates and synthetic colors and flavors. This sort of diet manipulation is technically known as an "elimination diet" because its only directive is to avoid certain forbidden items. All four children improved dramatically on this regimen. A boy named Michael Keyser, then aged seven, typified the first group. He had been cranky from birth, a fighter from the time he could walk, and had lived since age three and a half on a potent array of drugs intended to restrain his outbursts. Four years later, still adhering to Feingold's elimination plan, Michael needed no drugs, had been shifted to a normal classroom from one for "troubled" children, and had become, in the description of his mother, "an entirely different child. He's lovable, has a real sense of humor, and most of all, he likes himself."

Proceeding to treat hundreds of hyperactive children, Dr. Feingold found that up to half of them returned to normal or near-normal behavior when separated from the synthetic colors and flavors. His work received what could be termed its formal debut in a paper presented at the 1973 annual convention of the American Medical Association. By 1975, the FDA had reluctantly admitted there might "well be something to Feingold's research" and by 1977, several other researchers had attained findings that to a greater or lesser extent supported Dr. Feingold. This is not to say, however, that medicine basically accepts the Feingold thesis. A June 1978 "Commentary" in *Pediatrics* announced that "the evidence to date indicates that if there is a relationship between diet and behavior, it is either scarcely significant or it exists only among a small subpopulation of children." In the same issue of *Pediatrics* were two separate studies of the Feingold diet. The first, which concerned a group of 26 hyperactive children, reported that "there were clearly significant reductions [in hyperactive behavior] related to diet for approximately one-fourth of the children." The second study concerned two groups of children—36 school-age children and 10 three-to-five-year-olds. Although no consistent relation was found between diet and hyperactivity for the older children, all of the mothers and more than half the participating fathers of the younger children rated their children as greatly improved in behavior during the weeks they were on the diet.

Perhaps one reason that Dr. Feingold's work has been long in sinking in is that it embraces a complaint radically different in scope from the usual adverse finding about one food additive—a complaint that sweeps through the whole field of food protection like a swarm of avenging locusts, raising questions that promise to be more complex than any yet encountered. The American food supply, in an indulgence unmatched elsewhere in the world, is now home to some 3,000 different synthetic chemicals.

Moreover, it has usually been assumed that any price for this indulgence would be paid in physical form—in, for example, malignant cells or diseased livers. The creation of a distinct class of behavior-disturbed children was a novel possibility. Feingold likes to point out that the seeming emergence of hyperactivity as a modern plague paralleled an explosion in usage of the very chemicals he bans. The manufacture of synthetic food dyes, for example, almost doubled between 1960 and 1970, as marketing techniques saw foods as diverse as cereal, lunch meat, and baby preparations dyed almost neon in the competition for the customer's eye. Various official and semi-official estimates for hyperactivity also mounted steadily. As is often the case with behavior disorders, firm numbers are simply not to be had. But it has been claimed that as many as two to five million children have been sentenced to hyperactivity.

As time went by, experience with the Feingold diet tended to indict the colors and flavors even more seriously. Experience revealed, for example, that most children could tolerate the reintroduction of salicylates into their stomachs and lives, a tolerance that obviously pointed toward the colors and flavors as the primary provocateurs; it also simplified use of the diet. In most cases where the diet does help, parents need only worry about keeping their children away from the colors and flavors, rather than also having to regulate salicylates.

Experience also revealed that the effectiveness of the diet steadily diminished the older the child. Teenagers, for example, tend not to respond at all, or their improvement is spotty; by then, of course, it is possible that permanent damage has occurred. Age also tends to govern the length of time required for a child who does respond to the diet to clear his system of chemical intruders and retrieve control over his physical self. A Washington, D.C., pediatrician with some forty children on the diet describes watching some younger ones, those under five, "entirely change their personality in forty-eight hours." This doctor also prescribes the diet for children who are not "classically hyperactive, but just always whiny and cranky for what seems like no real reason." He finds it is often a great assist to them, too.

Older children may need a month to get going and an even longer period to overcome the psychological devastation imposed by their former, "bad" self. Accompanying sensorimotor deficits also tend to fade, again to an extent that depends on the age and condition of the child. An eleven-year-old child named David Hathaway once testified to this point at hearings before the health subcommittee of the Senate Labor and Public Welfare Committee. He said that, for him, the major benefit of the diet was his increased coordination. For the first time in his life, he could build model airplanes.

Perhaps the most impressive improvements are in children too hopeless to speak for themselves—those who suffer the double blow of behavior problems and known neurological damage—retarded and brain-injured children, and those with Down's syndrome. They will not ever be "normal," but with their behavior under control, many of them might well be able to lead lives outside institutions. Scattered reports suggest that the diet's impact on them is dazzling. For example, the Brant Sanitorium, an Ontario, Canada, home for retarded and handicapped children, tried the Feingold regimen on a profoundly retarded and endlessly violent eight-year-old boy and on a ten-year-old girl with meningmyelocele, a congenital condition that leaves the spinal cord exposed. The girl stopped the self-abusive tantrums during which she had scratched herself until she bled; the boy, according to a staff commentary, for the first time was able "to form relationships with Staff members . . . and is able to express affection."

In medical science, of course, the observations of a single physician are not considered proof of anything. It seemed that after Feingold's initial presentation to the AMA, his claims were destined for outright oblivion or, at best, semi-quack status. They garnered brief media attention and much clucking in *Prevention,* a magazine that serves as the *National Enquirer* of the American digestive tract. ("Are you listening, FDA? Is anybody listening?") But two years passed before the FDA encouraged other researchers to merely check his findings. And none of the half-dozen or so federal agencies with jurisdiction over foods, health, or children, which could have sponsored the long, costly controlled studies that do count as proof in science, was interested in Feingold—although some of these agencies have devoted millions of dollars to sponsoring studies that laud the use of drugs in hyperkinesis.

Dr. Feingold, however, was a remarkable and formidable opponent. He was endowed with abundant charm, upright posture, and lively brown eyes. He was driven by a conviction that food technology is scarring thousands of the young. And he was determined to force the Department of Health, Education and Welfare "to begin to help these parents understand they have some alternative to drugging their children." He launched a one-man campaign, giving interviews, guiding parents' groups, and lecturing. He wrote a book called *Why Your Child Is Hyperactive,* a chatty, anecdotal account of the discovery of the diet, which includes additive-free recipes supplied by his wife, Helene, a retired ballerina. But above all, Feingold treated hundreds of hyperactive children without charge. Whatever conventional medicine might say about him, the parents of these youngsters were willing to attempt almost anything to aid a child whom conventional medicine could only drug or ignore. Packing special lunches, baking homemade cookies, and reforming their food habits, they presented Feingold with an endless stream of success stories to present, in turn, to officials at HEW. (Not incidentally, these parents also found it easier than expected to wean their children from the candy-coated glories of an American childhood. Some kids do refuse to cooperate, but those who respond to the K-P regimen often feel so much better that they tend to police their own food. One satisfied six-year-old observed that his body "wasn't angry anymore.")

This combination of parental testimony and public pressure outraged the medical profession and even now it is hard to know whether it was the right tactic. Dr. Feingold chose to do it—rather than go the slow "proper" route of talking only to his colleagues and hoping for eventual studies—both because he was old and frankly wanted to make some progress with this matter before he died and because he was fully aware of the forces against him. To strike at toxic food additives, after all, is to strike at the nation's largest retail business. The influence of the food industry in protecting itself shows in the fact that many of the additives Feingold was talking about were, according to strict interpretation of the law, in the food supply illegally in the first place; and others were so toxic that common sense, if not the law, should have kept them out.

Feingold's complaints against food colors, for example, were basically directed against the so-called "coal-tar" dyes. First synthesized from coal in the 1850s and now made from oil, these additives have been continually controversial, whatever their raw base. The first one was banned in 1919. The technique has been for the government to ban with one hand those most recently found to be carcinogenic or toxic, and, with the other hand, to approve a slightly reformulated replacement from the same base. Although by now, in the phrase of Dr. Michael F. Jacobson, the Director of the Center for Science in the Public Interest, "the history of approved dyes reads like the guest register in a hotel for transients," the coal-tar colors remain the most commonly used dyes in the United States. Synthetic flavors, meanwhile, are a virtually unregulated class of additive. Some are said by industry to be "exact chemical copies" of natural flavors—or even better, "simplified chemical copies." Others contain chemicals that are variously used to manufacture antifreeze, paint remover, lice killer, cleaning fluids, and plastics. It is no wonder, John and Jan Jenkins have commented in *Environmental Action,* that "school custodians sometimes must use solvents to remove artificially flavored and colored ice cream that has hardened on lunch tables and chairs."

In the wake of Dr. Feingold, the National Institute of Education did finally allot funding to Dr. Keith Conners of the University of Pittsburgh for a brief, controlled study of fifteen children. Conners, a clinical psychologist who had been a leading figure in drugging hyperactive children—and occasionally a drug-company consultant—said later that he frankly had thought the diet would be quickly disproved. In a 1977 interview with the *Chicago Tribune,* he noted that he had opposed Feingold for years. "We were vigorous debating opponents on both TV and radio. But now I agree with some of his claims. My position changed last June when we completed a study in which children were daily fed chocolate chip cookies that looked and tasted alike. However, half contained artificial coloring and half did not. A small, but significant number of children showed definite hyperactive reactions to the food coloring."

Since then, some half-dozen published studies of hyperactivity and diet have supported Feingold to some degree. A few have not. The work most frequently cited against his thesis is the results with the older children in the two-part study just mentioned. Considering, however, that behavior studies are particularly difficult and expensive—and almost by necessity confined to small numbers of children—it is hardly surprising that their results are sometimes contradictory.

By now it is as well documented as many things in medicine that a discernible number of hyperactive children—if not a full 50 percent—respond to the Feingold regimen. To put it bluntly, Dr. Feingold's work is about a hundred-fold better documented than, say, the idea that "hormone supports" could prevent miscarriage ever was. And, on the off-chance that the supportive studies are in total error, there is—unlike using hormone supports—no danger to just trying out the diet on a distraught child for a few weeks to see what happens. There is a sense in which it may be confusing to even call the Feingold regimen a "diet." It is only food as food has traditionally been served through the ages—that is, without a plethora of additives, some of them barely tested at all, and others well known to be quite toxic. To Mrs. Carol Simone of Lawrence, Massachusetts, "It is really too bad that parents don't just try it before using drugs. There's no way you can harm your children. All you're giving them is good food. So what are you out?" Mrs. Simone's own son was prescribed an amphetamine-like drug for years. She and her husband turned to the diet for him when they became disturbed by the way the drug "just whacked him out."

✳

A half-dozen studies showing "varying degrees" of, say, liver damage, much less of cancer, in children who ate cookies loaded with artificial colors would never have languished the way these behavioral studies have. The government has literally not made a single regulatory move in response to them. There just seems to be something about behavior—and especially the behavior of children—that people have trouble accepting as a sign of toxicity. Maybe grownups find it hard to believe that a spanking or a psychiatrist or time itself can't bring all bad children around.

When used correctly, however, the term "hyperactive" does not describe young people who are merely naughty or just annoying. It describes children who are essentially as crippled in life as those who, because of physical injury, walk on crutches. Aside from the social crippling of being a "bad" child, many of these children also suffer from sensorimotor deficiencies. These difficulties in fine and gross motor control, in balance and eye focus, can render such school-related tasks as holding a pencil cruel obstacles. Like abused children, hyperactive children are thought to form a disproportionate number of the dropout and criminal young. The difference is that they have been flogged into a malign self-image by their own bodies.

Although hyperactivity seems to prefer blond, blue-eyed children, it marches indiscriminately across racial and social barriers. There is, however, general agreement that it affects boys some six times or more as often as girls. This could be a signal of genetic involvement or it could mean nothing more than the nursery-rhyme wisdom that boys, being made of puppy-dog tails, generally have more trouble growing up. There is also no general agreement about the true number of hyperactive children in the United States. As with many behavior disorders, the lack of a diagnostic test means that hyperactivity exists mainly in the eye of the beholder. The beholding of hyperactivity has ranged from the 2 percent or so of schoolchildren proposed a few years ago by the federal Office of Education to the 25 percent or more now claimed by some school districts. Skeptical observers suggest the term has lost its true meaning and become a catchall for any annoying or frantic behavior on the part of the young; and, in pediatrics, hyperactivity has something of a reputation as a "diagnostic garbage pail." In their 1975 book, sternly titled *The Myth of the Hyperactive Child,* Peter Schrag and Diane Divoky further propose that some groups, particularly the drug industry, which has been engaged in a frantic campaign to establish psychotropic medications as the modern solution for troublesome children, have a real stake in inflating the incidence of the disorder.

What seems most astonishing is that, for more than five years of controversy over Feingold, neither the FDA nor anyone else thought to simply behavior-test food colors or flavors on animals. Then, in 1978, a pediatric neurologist at Yale Medical School reported that young rats fed a mixture of food colors "contained in the average American diet" were unusually active and also had trouble performing certain standard tasks used to test learning ability.

It is perhaps symptomatic of the human problem in dealing with behavioral toxicity that these rat tests have now impressed some people more than all the previous reports of improved conduct in real children put on the Feingold diet. "Just when I had hoped the Feingold diet could be put into the same category as the apple-a-day," Dr. Sydney Gellis commented in *Pediatric Notes,* the weekly newsletter he edits, "this study appears and will greatly strengthen the Feingold forces. We shall now have to go back to square one and start all over again because in these times you can't disregard animal studies. I don't like this one bit!"

Feingold's work emerged simultaneously with a cluster of similar observations about other environmental agents. Taken alone, these discoveries might not have made much of a public or medical impression; taken together, they suggest there is hardly a limit to the things that can steal like nightmare across young minds.

A report from McGill University in Montreal, Canada, is especially interesting. A research group there came across the "quite unexpected" finding that, by measuring the trace metal content of children's hair, they could predict with 98 percent accuracy whether teacher rating scales and standardized tests would characterize a particular child as "learning disabled." This correlation between the body burden of certain trace elements—the ones measured were cadmium, cobalt, magnesium, chromium, and lithium—and learning problems does not necessarily mean that trace metals cause such problems. That may or may not be true in individual cases. More important, the "unexpected finding" at McGill again underlines that children differ individually in their ability to metabolize chemicals. As the general chemical load increases, more and more may find themselves generally in trouble because their bodies cannot keep up with the task.

The New York Institute of Child Development, a nonprofit center in Manhattan whose staff is much interested in the physiology of behavior disturbances, is also a rich source of revealing incidents. Over the years, by analyzing factors ranging from the glucose tolerance of individual children to their general diets and the trace metal content of their hair, the Institute staff has identified youngsters who regained their composure when separated from items as diverse as cow's milk and copper. "No matter how long you work in this field," comments William Mullineaux, the Institute's former clinical director, "you are still astonished by what some of the most common things will do to a child whose system can't handle them."

To illustrate this point, the Institute staff likes to tell the story of two eight-year-olds brought to them simultaneously. One child was a sunny, blond boy whom the staff nicknamed "Adorable Arthur" in honor of how really good he was when good. Yet, for all his charm, Arthur had occasional fits in which he smashed anything, human or object, within reach. Detective work correlating his rages to his appetite revealed that Arthur's parents had not understood that apples were included among the salicylate fruits forbidden to this boy. For the other angry eight-year-old, however, apples were a fortunate fruit. He was suffering from an excessive ingestion of copper—an excess that perhaps was taken in with his drinking water. A daily half cup of homemade apple sauce (an overprocessed commercial brand would not have worked) served as a natural chelating agent to draw out the offending chemical.

The contemporary world, however, is not marked just by chemical pollution, but by the use of physical devices—from microwaves to fluorescent lighting—that may equally harass the nervous system. Dr. John Ott, founder of the Environmental Health and Light Research Institute in Fort Lauderdale, Florida, a few years ago tried an experiment that involved changing the lighting source for first-graders assigned to windowless classrooms in the Sarasota, Florida, school system. He replaced their "Cool White" tubes with "Full Spectrum" fluorescent tubes designed to closely simulate natural outdoor light. He also shielded these tubes to block the electromagnetic radiation that escapes from virtually all fluorescents.

Dr. Ott's primary interest was in the behavior of the children. He reported in the journal *Eye, Ear, Nose and Throat* that teachers in the Full Spectrum classrooms felt the "overall classroom performance" of the children had substantially improved. They were no longer endlessly engaged in the sort of fidgety behavior—sprawling on desks, careening in their chairs, and banging around—that seems to have become the hallmark of American classrooms. Dr. Ott also backed this behavior observation with a physical one. Young rodents raised under Cool White fluorescents develop more cavities than rodents raised under Full Spectrum tubes. Ott asked a team of dentists to check whether this curious circumstance would also hold for young humans. By the end of the school year, half the first-graders in Cool-White classrooms had cavities in their six-year molars. Under the Full Spectrum tubes, fewer than one quarter did.

✳

There is one substance above all that has underscored the difficulty in coming to terms with environmentally induced behavior problems. That substance is lead, the single most studied chemical known. Observers from the ancient Greeks to Benjamin Franklin have remarked its poisonous nature. (Although the ancient Romans seemed to have known about lead toxicity, they nonetheless made such great use of lead utensils and implements that some theorize that widespread brain damage helped bring down the Roman Empire.) Lead poisoning among industrial workers was a well-understood disease by the nineteenth century. By comparison, other chemicals are mere baubles of research and babes in the toxicology lab. It is a major lesson that even with all this study, even today, fresh and serious revelations about lead's impact on children are still coming in almost like shock waves. In 1979, in the blunt estimation of Dr. Vernon Houk, the Director of Environmental Services at the Center for Disease Control in Atlanta, lead toxicity among young children still remains "the number one or two public health problem in large areas of the United States."

The insight that the pastimes of childhood pose a great risk for lead exposure originally came from the unlikely place of Queensland, Australia, the state that occupies the northeastern wedge of that continent. In the 1890s, Queensland found itself in the middle of a seething lead epidemic, with some 200 of its children each year succumbing to the seizures, cramps, and paralysis typical of severe lead poisoning. There seemed to be no explanation at all. The place was barely settled, much less industrialized, and certain aspects of the epidemic only darkened the mystery. Why weren't other areas of Australia affected? Why, with the source being ubiquitous enough to strike down several hundred children, were adults entirely spared and why, most of all, was the poisoning most evident in the middle-class children of the towns while few rural children became sick? Frantic study of water supplies, of food containers, and of any number of possible lead sources failed to identify the source. Finally, in 1904, in a classic of epidemiology published in the *Australian Medical Gazette* under the title "A Plea for Painted Railings and Painted Walls of Rooms as the Source of Lead Poisoning among Queensland Children," Dr. J. Lockhart Gibson pierced the ugly secret. The paint then in use in Queensland contained about 70 percent lead, and children had become its victims because they tend to chew whatever they encounter on the floor, including paint dust and chips.

There was a sense in which the children of Queensland were victims of the taste and wealth of their parents. Because of Queensland's pounding sun and torrid days, airy verandahs, painted white from floorboard to ceiling, had become a popular addition to its town houses. These verandahs, where young children would be set out to play, were the primary source of lead. Even from almost a century's distance, it is hard not to feel the poignancy of the Queensland epidemic—not to see, in the mind's eye, young mothers setting out their children in what looked to be pleasant, protected places but what were really poisonous, over-sized cribs. Rural children had been spared because their parents could not afford to build and paint verandahs.

Having discovered the first real environmental epidemic of childhood, medical science immediately marched forward to make the calamitous, if natural, error of assuming an exact analogy to biological disease. If polio was accompanied by fever and measles by spots, lead poisoning was accompanied by nausea, headaches, and cramps. Unfortunately, by the time these "symptoms" appear, the child might well be headed toward death or toward lead encephalopathy. The combined product of damage to the nerve cells and edema of the brain, severe encephalopathy, in the unsentimental phrase of one commentator, often leaves behind "total mental defectives with no hope of return to normal activity."

Socially, the concept of lead poisoning as an "overt" disease made it seem a rare occurrence brought on by doses larger than those usually encountered in food, water, and air. Medically, the concept of overt disease precluded people from thinking that chemicals might have an attack pattern quite different from, say, viruses—a pattern of low-level assaults that did not produce much in the way of symptoms until, too late, the cumulative damage showed itself. The history of lead poisoning has essentially been a history of trying to destroy these two concepts; and, while many doctors and public health officials have actually long recognized lead as a poison causing rather widespread central nervous system damage at quite low levels of ingestion, it has not been easy for them to bring their colleagues around to their thinking. In a world of a thousand lead objects, both the medical and popular mind had early seized on paint chips as the "extraordinary" source that must account for most lead poisoning. This notion has been so firmly believed that the *New York Times*, in its annual index, listed—and still lists—lead-poisoning stories, not under the heading "lead," but under the heading "paints." And, in the United States, the association with paint chips essentially worked to make lead poisoning seem a disease solely of the slums and carelessness, and neglected children who went around eating things off the floor. This notion was so firmly held that, in a 1970 pamphlet, the Department of Health, Education and Welfare described the disease as being "prevalent only among children whose families are least able to improve their living conditions. The well-informed segments of the population," HEW blandly reassured, "are seldom affected."

A couple of years later, however, when the federal government began to test children routinely for lead poisoning, no one was reassured. Even in the wealthy reaches of Westchester County, the suburban pride of New York, some 5 percent of children surveyed had, if not outright poisoning, then definite "excess" lead ingestion. And, in a few more years, the news would be even more discomforting. By then, several researchers had shown that measurable numbers of children were sustaining central nervous system damage—these children were fidgety and hyperactive, sometimes retarded and frequently just not able to cooperate in school, whatever their IQ—at levels of lead ingestion well below those even today officially considered to represent "excess" lead ingestion in the young.

*

Every revolution has an arbitrary date at which accumulated grievances burst forth. A date for the beginning of the revolution in medical attitudes toward lead might be set at the fall 1973 publication in the *New England Journal of Medicine* of a two-part series by Dr. Jane Lin-Fu called "Vulnerability of Children to Lead Exposure and Toxicity." Ironically, it had been Dr. Lin-Fu who had, as a pediatric consultant to HEW, a few years earlier penned the belief that lead rarely assaulted "the well-informed segments of the population." In those few years, she and other people had become very disenchanted with the conventional wisdom that lead's dangers lay in high doses, overt symptoms, and slum conditions.

By the late 1960s those few cities whose health departments were then concerned about lead at all were reporting that 20 to 40 percent of the poisoned children coming to their attention did not have a verified history of ingesting paint or plaster chips. This fact pointed toward other lead sources as contributing to poisoning. For young children, whose mouths are full participants in their exploration of the world, daily life presents endless lead sources that adults need not fear. Children munch lead on toothpaste tubes, suck it off pencils, and chew it off newspapers. (Printer's ink has a substantial lead content.) It is, however, the use of lead as an antiknock additive to gasoline that has really made it a toxin from which there is no place to hide. Between 1935 and 1976, the amount of lead added to gasoline rose from 37,000 to 240,000 tons. By the late 1960s, Dr. Lin-Fu pointed out, so much lead was spewing from America's tailpipes and coming to rest on playgrounds or inside houses that, in some urban areas, a child need swallow only $1/24$ teaspoon of local dirt or house dust to exceed the recommended daily lead intake for young children.

Scientists had also belatedly realized that lead acts differently and far more dangerously inside the bodies of children than of adults. While adults simply excrete most of the lead they swallow or breathe in, children absorb about 40 percent of the amount that enters their bodies. Of the small amount of lead they do take in, adults send about 90 percent straight to the bones where it binds itself, a permanent guest in the skeleton assumed to cause no harm. Children under age six, by contrast, send only about two-thirds of their body burden of lead to the bones; the rest continues to wander ominously through the blood and soft tissues. And even then, the younger the child, evidently the worse can be the damage from this wandering lead. The first ten postnatal days of neural development in the rat approximate the first two and a half years of human life; it requires only one-quarter the amount of lead to cause the same stunting of learning abilities in one-to-ten-day-old rats as in rats eleven days old or more.

Medical scientists, then, had long misunderstood both the sources of lead reaching children and its distribution once inside young bodies. Lin-Fu wondered whether something else had also been profoundly misunderstood—namely, lead's true effects. When children are frankly lead poisoned, there is no question but that they can sustain permanent and far-reaching damage. Follow-up of such children ten to forty years afterward has brought forth adults with any number of dreary complaints; they have kidney disease, gouty arthritis, mental retardation, and psychological disturbances. But what of the long-term prospects for children not frankly lead poisoned, yet with blood lead levels above those considered normal or average? In the United States, this is a prodigious number of children; in the years since the federal government has sponsored wide-scale screening, about 5 to 10 percent of the children annually tested have had "undue" amounts of lead in their blood. In 1973, there had been so little study of the fate of these children that Dr. Lin-Fu was forced to end her series in the *New England Journal of Medicine* with a question—one of the most crucial public health questions ever posed. "Is the vulnerability of young children to this lethal element," she asked, "such that subtle, yet irreversible damage is being sustained by those with undue lead absorption, but not considered to be lead poisoned according to current criteria?"

*

In 1972, the federal Childhood Lead Control Program had used a blood lead level of 40 micrograms (a microgram is one-thousandth of a gram and often abbreviated as mcg) per 100 milliliters (ml) of blood as the level officially considered to represent "undue" or "excess" lead absorption in young children. Children with this level were not necessarily to be treated—indeed children with a blood lead level of 40 mcg are not often treated even today—but they were to be watched in case their level ascended further, and some effort was to be made to find the source of their lead absorption and remove it from their lives if possible.

Barely had the government set the 40 mcg level than there came the first strong hint that thousands of young minds could well be lost to that very amount of lead. In a study published in the *Journal of Pediatrics* in 1972, Dr. Brigitte de la Burdé, a Richmond, Virginia, pediatrician, followed the development of children who as toddlers had had fairly brief bouts of lead ingestion that had brought their blood lead levels above 40 mcg, but who had never been considered to be lead poisoned or to have displayed symptoms that would call for treatment. Testing the children when they were four years old showed that deviations in "overall behavior ratings occurred almost three times as often in children with lead exposure compared to the control subjects. The most frequent combination of behavior characteristics was extreme negativism, distractibility and constant need for attention."

And, as time went by, even though their blood lead continued to be normal, the aftermath of their early lead exposure became more obvious and more distressing. Evaluation of them at ages seven and eight showed "severe behavior problems at home (lying, stealing, running away, fire setting) in fourteen lead-exposed children as compared to six control children. . . . Five lead-exposed children had been seen by psychiatrists, one has since been institutionalized, and three were receiving treatment for seizures. Fifteen lead-exposed children had made poor academic progress compared to two controls."

"Most of the children who failed in school," Dr. Burdé pointed out in the October, 1975, *Journal of Pediatrics,* "had an average IQ at seven years. School failure in many of these students was due to behavioral problems interfering with learning. Nineteen lead-exposed children were described as hyperactive, impulsive and explosive, and as having frequent temper tantrums."

Overall, about 20 percent of the lead-exposed children seem to have been severely cut down by the time they were three years old, with school failure, seizures, psychiatrists, and even institutionalization being their destined lot—although no one knew it at the time. What added to Burdé's observations was that, during the years she was studying and reporting on this group of Richmond children, the federal Childhood Lead Control Program was uncovering literally thousands of children who, to judge from their blood levels, stood in the same realm of risk.

In 1972, under the auspices of the Childhood Lead Control Program, the United States had become the first Western nation to monitor—and sometimes even treat—lead absorption among a good percentage of its children each year. At about the same time, the federal government also strengthened controls on lead in gasoline, food containers, and other products. With these tactics, the United States did achieve real leadership in lead control. And, on one level, the results have been gratifying: it has been shown that a severe environmental epidemic can, like the severe biological epidemics of the past, be contained and treated. Both childhood deaths from lead poisoning and cases of severe lead encephalopathy are now very rare.

Still, on another level, the Childhood Lead Program was severely distressing. As the government began to systematically test children, it became obvious that the lead problem was simply out of control. During the first three years of its operations, when a blood lead level of 40 mcg or more was defined as "undue" lead absorption, some 6½ percent of the more than one million children under age six screened by the program exceeded this level. In 1975, "undue" lead absorption was redefined as a blood level of 30 mcg or more. By 1978, the last full year for which figures are available, almost 7 percent of the 400,000 children tested still had undue absorption and 2 percent stood in the very dangerous zone of 50 mcg or more. Not only did thousands and thousands of children have too high a body burden of lead, but lead toxicity had become a leading childhood disease in the United States. Its age-specific attack rate of 140 per 100,000, reported the Center for Disease Control, "exceeds the rates reported for most childhood diseases."

It was also evident that, even with sincere efforts to curb lead use, thousands of children would continue to display these levels for years to come. The stuff is just so woven into the fabric of industrialized life that, even as one source, such as paint chips, is partially confronted, another seems to crop up to take its place. Recent worry, for example, has focused on lead corrosion from water pipes installed decades ago and now starting to deteriorate.

The next question was proper treatment for these thousands of lead-exposed children suddenly being found all across the country. At present, the standard treatment for lead ingestion involves administering a chelating agent, which binds to the lead, drawing it out for excretion. This is done with a five-day series of painful injections or with pills administered over several weeks. Chelation requires that children be closely watched—sometimes they are hospitalized—on the chance that they might react adversely to the agent itself or to lead "mobilized" from the bones for removal. Simply to subject thousands of children to chelation without some clinical evidence of benefit to each child would not be medically proper. The trouble is that individual responses to lead vary so notoriously it is not easy to say which children really need chelation.

The great quest in lead toxicology, as Dr. Julian Chisolm, the pioneering American lead researcher, once put it, has been to find "a sensitive and specific biological change" that could detect the first signs that an individual child was faltering because of lead— and detect this faltering before permanent damage occurred. At present, the measurement of erythrocyte protoporphyrin (EP) is as close as there is to such a "specific biological change." Erythrocyte protoporphyrin, which is a precursor of hemoglobin, builds up in the blood at the point where lead interferes in the formation of the heme portion of red blood cells. Too much interference in hemoglobin synthesis leaves the child anemic. There is a general feeling that EP may be "the best we can do now" to try to get at individual responses to lead; but there is also concern that EP still does not say what is happening to brain cells. Blood is available for testing; brain cells, of course, are not. The irony is that the blood will regenerate itself and overcome anemia after lead is removed; a brain cell destroyed, however, is a brain cell gone forever.

By the mid-1970s, evidence was accumulating that even a blood lead level of 30 mcg was not always low enough. In 1975, for example, a Glasgow, Scotland, research group had reported that the mean blood lead level of a group of retarded four-and-a-half-year-olds was 25.5 mcg; for control children who were not retarded, the mean blood lead level stood at 18.7 mcg. At the same time, work in the United States took an indictment of lead down to this very small amount.

Dr. Oliver David, a tall, bearded psychiatrist, is the director of the Child Behavior Unit at Downstate Medical Center, an institution located in the Flatbush section of Brooklyn, New York. Nearby, brisk street names like State and Winthrop clash oddly with the debris-strewn sidewalks and children seem to be in a lot of trouble all around. At the Child Behavior Unit, there is Christopher, exuberant in red sneakers, who is brought in by an older sister. She describes him as "never doing nothing right." There is Tyrone, who is possessed of a charming and confused smile and who has been put back a grade in school. His mother is "not too happy" with Tyrone.

Dr. David had found himself "constantly bothered in trying to apply conventional psychiatric explanations" to the troubles of many of these children and had, among other things, begun to wonder whether low-level lead might be responsible for some of their behavior. First, by taking two groups of children, he investigated a link with hyperactivity. One group had a probable medical cause that could explain their hyperactive behavior—for instance, a difficult or premature birth, which could have left slight brain damage—and the second group had "no probable cause." The mean blood lead levels of these groups proved to be slightly but significantly different—22.9 versus 26.2 mcg. The two groups also differed in their response to several weeks of chelation. There was no general improvement in the behavior of the "probable cause" children; but, David reported in the October, 1976, *American Journal of Psychiatry*, with the lowering of their blood lead, five out of seven of the "no probable cause" children were judged by teachers, parents, and doctors alike to have shown a "widespread improvement in behavior." With this two-group approach, David had been able to demonstrate two important principles—namely that hyperactivity *per se* is not a cause of increased lead absorption, and that the chelation therapy had not functioned as a placebo. Only children with raised blood lead levels had responded to it. Moreover, as had the Glasgow results, David's children suggested what fearfully small amounts of lead may stand between normalcy and abnormalcy.

Dr. David next used this two-group approach to compare mentally retarded children; as with hyperactive children, he found a difference in blood lead levels between mentally retarded children with a "probable cause" for their retardation and those whose retardation was without known cause—in this case, 18.7 mcg versus 25.5 mcg. There was, however, no point to chelating the retarded children. If lead were responsible for their condition, removing it would not improve their minds; any damage of that sort was already permanent.

Not surprisingly, Dr. David considers the whole concept of trying to name threshold levels for "excess" lead absorption— whether the government officially chooses to set the level at 40 mcg or 30 mcg or even 25—as "an absurdity. The correct thing," he argues, "would be to talk about a continuum of effects. I would say that it would be rare to find a child with noticeable damage below 20 micrograms, but even then you have no guarantee there isn't some decrement in the child's abilities." Dr. David also likes to emphasize that chelation is hardly the same as a cure. Even when done at the first slight signs of neurological stress, it may prevent further damage, but it can hardly erase damage that may have already occurred. There is precisely one cure for lead toxicity and that is to keep the stuff out of the environment in the first place.*

Still, the idea of "low-level" lead toxicity did not gain firm acceptance until March 1979. It was then that Dr. Herbert L. Needleman and a research team at Children's Hospital Medical Center in Boston published their astounding investigation of widespread problems of behavior and school performance in first- and second-graders, living in the towns of Chelsea and Somerville on the edge of Boston, who had sustained "symptomless" lead ingestion. Two factors gave the Needleman study particular weight. In the first place, by focusing on lead injury to a population of white children living in towns, it may have finally slain the notion that lead is only a real threat to black children who live in ghettos. In the second place, the Needleman group did not analyze the children's blood lead levels, but instead studied the lead content of their teeth. Blood lead levels are a transient measure. Lead, however, binds permanently to the teeth, as it does to other parts of the skeletal system. As their baby teeth fell out, the children were asked to bring them in for study; and, in somewhat the fashion that rings on the trunk of a tree reveal its age, the lead content of these young teeth confirmed that many

---

* In a letter he wrote to *Pediatrics* a few years ago, Dr. David pointed out another, perhaps important, factor in contemporary lead toxicity. He expressed his surprise at having learned that EDTA, a chemical long favored in medicine as a chelating agent, is also "used ubiquitously as a food additive." EDTA's job in food is about the same as its job in children—to bind metals. In a huge range of products—mayonnaise, processed fruits, and beer alike—it neutralizes the metal scrapings that creep into food during its journey through the rollers, blenders, and bins of the modern processing line. "The amount used as an additive," David commented, "is sufficient to cause some lead mobilization, but not sufficient to effect a definitive 'deleading.' " In other words, EDTA in food might well nudge enough lead from the bones to cause some trouble on its own or, at the least, to cause trouble in association with other sources of lead.

children in Somerville and Chelsea had long-standing lead exposures.

The higher the lead concentration in the children's teeth, the
lower they scored on a battery of intelligence and functional tests
and the lower their teachers rated their behavior and cooperation.
The first subtle impact of lead seemed to be felt in the child's
ability to concentrate, and from there, language and organizational
skills went downhill. The children with high lead concentrations in
their teeth often had trouble following simple directions; they
were overly active and impulsive. They "performed significantly
less well on the Wechsler Intelligence scale, particularly the verbal
items, on three measures of auditory and verbal processing, on
attentional performance as measured by reaction time under
conditions of varying delay and on most items of the teachers'
behavioral rating," the Needleman group commented.

Still, high lead dentine concentrations as defined in Chelsea
and Somerville did not mean levels generally considered dangerous. No child studied had ever been suspected of lead toxicity.
The only information about their previous blood lead levels came
from a local program, through which some had once been tested as
preschoolers. The mean blood lead level of these old tests stood at
35.5 mcg—a level that, a few years ago, did not officially represent
"undue" lead absorption and that, even today, would rarely if ever
be considered a call for chelation.

The main sources of lead exposure in Chelsea and Somerville
are not fully known. Only 30 percent of the most affected children
were said to have had pica—a prolonged and noticeable habit of
eating nonfood items—when they were very young. Those who
happened to live in homes with old, peeling paint may have
consumed a lot of paint chips in their toddler days, but the rest
may just have accumulated it from various sources; a few paint
chips here and there, perhaps; constant small amounts from the
exhaust of local traffic; some in the water supply and some in food
containers. This is again a reminder of the practical limits of
chelation. Can the nation tolerate widespread lead exposures that
might require that 5 percent or more of its young children be

routinely chelated in order to prevent them from later performing "significantly less well" in school and in life?

Queensland, Australia, had launched lead poisoning as a middle-class disease; it had taken Chelsea and Somerville—and seventy-five years—to finally bring it home as a middle-class reality.

During the past decade and a half, as everyone who worries about the future knows, young people and teenagers have been committing unprecedented numbers of violent crimes, while the intellectual performance of American high school graduates, as measured by the National Scholastic Aptitude Test (SAT), has declined steadily. These are obviously complex trends; in 1977, a special panel of the College Entrance Examination Board cited lowered teaching standards, more divorce, television watching, and "unprecedented turbulence in the nation's affairs" as among the possible reasons for the scholastic decline. It seems equally likely, however, that the physical environment has added in some measure to these national worries; it does not take much foresight to see that Dr. Burdé's "impulsive and explosive" children, Dr. David's retarded children, and Dr. Feingold's hyperactive children are bound to turn up in someone's statistics eventually, whether those of the SAT or of their local police department.

To actually quantify the environmental role in severe disorders of learning and behavior is, however, probably impossible. Still, people do attempt it. One place where this attempt is being made is the Full Circle School in Bolinas, California. Founded in 1974 by Michael Lerner, a young psychologist, the Full Circle School deals with violent, disturbed, and criminal children—many of whom come directly there from juvenile detention centers. As Lerner had suspected that many such children were as ill physically as they might be disturbed psychologically, the first group was given detailed physical, psychological, and neurological examinations. The extent of ill health among these sad children and teenagers surprised even a staff who had surmised they would be in poor shape. All of them had severe eye or perceptual problems. The most violent one, a sixteen-year-old who assaulted the counselors "on numerous occasions," was so hypoglycemic that he hallucinated; another boy had such severe convulsions that he lost consciousness three times a day. But, among all their physical ills, what most stood out was a range of allergies and sensitivities so severe that one wonders whether these young people had ever felt quite normal or comfortable for a day in their lives.

Dr. Clyde Hawley, a Livermore, California, allergist, tested the children for food and chemical reactions. Dr. Hawley did not bother with anything so esoteric as baking them little cookies with hidden additives; he simply used the standard allergy techniques of sublingual (placing a test substance under the tongue) and subcutaneous (injecting a drop of a substance under the skin) testing. Food dyes, for instance, were tested sublingually. The following summarizes Hawley's findings about six children:

A. (Black male, age 10, hyperactive with a severe learning disability and a history of violence.) Was hyperactive on phenol [a chemical with various uses sometimes found, for instance, in tin can linings and disinfectants]. Red food dye caused an extreme positive reaction and A became very belligerent. Blue food dye made him even more belligerent. He threw things around the office. Yellow food dye made him roll on the floor. He was irritable on corn; wheat caused some depression.

B. (White male, age 14, small for his age, with a learning disability and a history of violence.) Became very tired on red food dye and had a probable positive reaction to cane sugar.

C. (White male, age 16, with a learning disability, a history of extreme violence and hypoglycemia.) He was irritable on red dye. Wheat depressed him and he looked pale. Milk made him feel very disoriented and beef made him grumpy. His hands trembled on yeast.

D. (Black male, age 12, with a severe learning disability and a history of violence.) Synthetic alcohol made him very sleepy.

[Synthetic alcohol generally measures the response to petro-chemical products, including oil and gas fumes.] Wheat gave him a runny nose. Milk and yeast made him angry. Beet sugar produced hyperactivity. Red food dye made him sleepy but talkative and restless. Blue was a questionable positive, as was yellow.

E. (White male, age 11, extremely hyperactive, with a learning disability. Violent and subject to epileptiform seizures during rage.) He was sleepy on synthetic alcohol, irritable and hyperactive on corn and wheat. Milk caused a flush but no behavior change. Red food dye caused a very strong positive response. He became very angry and would not respond to questions. His throat was swollen and hoarse for hours after the food color tests.

F. (White male, age 11, extremely hyperactive with a learning disability, general disorientation, and visual hallucinations suggestive of organic damage.) He had an extremely severe response to egg; he became flushed and extremely dis-oriented. Wheat caused a similar but less severe response. He also became hyperactive on yeast. He was agitated on red food dye and belligerent on blue. Blue also made him tired, however, and he lay down on the clinic floor. Yellow caused a flush and hyperactivity. He talked continuously for three hours after the food color tests.

It was not, by the way, news to Dr. Hawley that a ten-year-old given a few drops of diluted food dye would start throwing things around the office and rolling on the floor. Hawley is one of the hard core of clinical allergists who have been treating troubled children on this basis for years. "I've seen hundreds of these children by now," he says, "and it doesn't surprise me at all!" In his experience, the coal-tar dyes are by far the worst offenders against children, followed by the sugars—corn, cane, and beet. He estimates that about 60 percent of troubled children improve greatly after intervention in their diet, that another 20 percent improve somewhat, and the rest just do not respond to this sort of treatment. He also believes that "you have to get them young. Otherwise, it often just doesn't work."

At Full Circle, all the six violent and allergy-prone children were put on diets free of synthetic colors and flavors. This tactic, Michael Lerner has written, helped "considerably—and in some cases dramatically." But, he cautions, "saying food additives alone are the most significant allergic factor in their disorders would be to simplify the picture considerably. While allergic factors are often of primary importance, particularly in behavior disorders, they are also often only symptomatic of more generalized underlying disorders to be diagnosed and tested."

None of the people working with the environmental causes of behavior disorders regard, say, dietary intervention or deleading as a magic prescription for happy children. Life is too complex for that, children are too complex, and the brain, also, is too complex. Michael Lerner still considers an old-fashioned "loving home" to be the first ingredient of juvenile happiness. Dr. Lendon Smith, whose *Improving Your Child's Behavior Chemistry* is a lucid guide for families with troubled children—and one many doctors would also profit by reading—still considers that the nutrients available to the brain when it is forming are as important as natural and chemical antagonists the child may encounter in later life.

But it is discouraging for people working on the environment and behavior to see children automatically drugged, time after time, without the least attention to alternatives. The drugging question is not fully black or white. Even people trying hard to find other ways to help these children may sometimes find themselves the reluctant users of drugs. "On the one hand," comments Dr. David, "we have a drug we know will work now whose future disadvantages are unknown; on the other hand, we have a kid who has been kicked out of school, who is constantly attacked by other kids, and who may be crippled for life if something isn't done."

Still, putting thousands of young children on amphetamines is a mass experiment in itself—and one that may carry heavy consequences. Past experience with drugs, of course, promises that "unexpected" side effects are just what should reasonably be expected. Already it is known that children on amphetamines do not grow properly. Their growth slows, and then, when the drug is taken away, undergoes a huge "catch-up" spurt. More ominously, it was reported in 1973 that patients with Hodgkin's disease, a cancer of the lymphatic system, include unusual numbers of people who have been prolonged and heavy users of amphetamines. This finding does not necessarily mean that amphetamines "cause" Hodgkin's disease; it could be the drug just hastens the appearance of malignancies already there. The strength of the link between amphetamines and Hodgkin's disease was, however, so surprising to the original research team that they decided to investigate another group of patients. Completed in early 1979, this second effort confirmed the amphetamine link. "I definitely think," comments Ruth Dworsky, a researcher at the University of Southern California School of Medicine who participated in both projects, "that we should now set up some animal work to see if we can find out what's really happening."

Yet, even if amphetamines—drugs considered so potent that it is a felony to obtain them without a prescription—could be proven perfectly safe stuff for three-, four-, and five-year-olds, they would still hardly be a solution to behavioral problems. To the extent that these problems are environmental, masking their symptoms with drugs is not any more clever than claiming to cure cancer by masking the pain. On a mass scale, such drugging may disguise important clues to environmental messes in the making; it is interesting, for example, that among all the maladies of the Love Canal children—their deafness, birth defects, respiratory disease, and seizures—the perhaps most consistent complaint of parents was that the behavior of their children was so out of control. And, on an individual basis, such drugging may just disguise that the child is sustaining severe and permanent damage from a central nervous system toxin, such as lead. The tragedy is that it can be so easy to diagnose the causes of individual distress; physicians are using amphetamines in preference to the simple steps of trying an elimination diet for a few weeks, testing the child's reaction to natural allergens, and screening the child for lead absorption (a process that requires sending all of four drops of blood to the laboratory). Perhaps nowhere else in medicine has the line been so tightly drawn between those physicians trying to understand environmental disease and those who have simply declined to deal with the new dangers of the age.

The government has also substantially joined in the refusal to deal with behavioral toxins. Only eight days after the *New England Journal of Medicine* published Needleman's jolting report on lead toxicity among the children of Somerville and Chelsea—and an accompanying editorial, which declared it to be "abundantly clear that undue lead absorption is matched by few other pediatric health problems"—the Carter Administration announced that its new "energy package" would include a relaxation of previously scheduled reductions in the lead content of gasoline. Controlling toxic food additives seems even more of a challenge. The world of "hard science" is so suspicious of behavior as a toxic signal that possibly only linking various food additives to physical disorders will force a change. Dr. Ott was able to identify tooth decay as the physical complaint that reinforced his observations about some fluorescent lights; the Feingold diet may well find similar reinforcement in eye disorders. As time passes and more families use the diet, some have occasionally begun to report marked improvement in the eyesight of their children.

One of these children is a boy named Michael Simone, who lives in Lawrence, Massachusetts. He was born with nystagmus, a disorder in which the eyeballs are subject to constant involuntary movement; they could be said to twitch. At age five, Michael's vision was 20/300, and when he went to school, he could only learn to read by using special large-type books. Because of the special books and his twitching eyes, he was often teased into tears by the other children. Michael was also hyperactive and had been prescribed an amphetamine-like drug when he started school. Three years later, more and more disturbed by this drug use, his parents decided to try the Feingold diet. In three days, they noticed that his behavior was remarkably better; but three months later, to their total astonishment, they also noticed that the nystagmoid movements of Michael's eyeballs had decreased and that he had backed away from his usual spot a few feet in front of the TV set. "We were shocked, as a matter of fact," Carol Simone recalls. "When I called up my ophthalmologist, I think he thought I was crazy."

The ophthalmologist, Dr. Jerome Crampton, may not have thought Mrs. Simone was crazy, but he was skeptical. However, when he reevaluated Michael's eyes and found that the child's vision was 20/80, he and the Simones decided on a little test to determine whether the diet was really responsible for the improvement. They let Michael eat junk food again for three days. Within that time, his vision deteriorated right back to 20/300. Again on the diet, Michael quickly recovered his 20/80 vision and, some months later, his vision stood at 20/50. "I don't know what this means in general," comments Dr. Crampton, "but I can say that in this one case, the nystagmus lessened very much when the child's diet was restricted."

Individual diets, however, are neither a fair nor a proper answer for dealing with toxins that are in the general food supply and within the constant reach of children. Sooner or later, there has to be a decision. Will a public accustomed from birth to forty-eight flavors, to Count Chocula cereal, and to coloring its food with known carcinogens give up some of these delights for a group of disturbed children whose numbers are so uncertain it cannot be said for sure whether they should be counted by the thousands or the millions? How many children are worthy the pink frosting on the cake?

Since DES I've thought about it and thought about it and as far as I can tell, man is the only animal who takes risks when he doesn't have to. Of course, other animals take risks. But they do it for a reason—to get food or to protect their young. Sometimes I don't think we'll get anywhere with the environment until we understand why man takes these risks for no reason.

DR. HOWARD ULFELDER

# Chapter 5

# CANCER BEFORE BIRTH

On a clear May day in 1971, Laurie Sale, a housewife in Watertown, Massachusetts, picked up the morning *Boston Globe* and felt herself almost assaulted by the front page. There, under the headline "Rare Cancer Linked to Synthetic Hormone," was the first public report of the carcinogenicity of DES. "The compound, called stilbestrol," the *Globe* reported, "was used fairly widely in Boston from 1946 to 1951 to help prevent miscarriages. It fell into disfavor after that and has been used very little in the past fifteen years." Mrs. Sale, a pretty, red-haired woman, was then in the eighth month of her second pregnancy. Her doctor had prescribed and she had taken the "disfavored" compound. A month later, she gave birth to a little girl, and has since then lived with a "psychological reality," as she explains it, perhaps not quite comprehensible to those not in its grip. "The bottom line," she says, "is that you can be told about your own daughter's risk ratio in a general sense and you can be told that only three hundred women out of thousands have developed cancer, and yet you've got a panicked population. The difference is that there's something that has affected my daughter's body over which I have no control. It's not like smoking. She can't give it up."

If Mrs. Sale felt herself assaulted, so did much of biological science. DES was not just a matter of a drug's causing cancer, but the vanguard in a profound, even revolutionary reappraisal of cancer causation. As late as 1970, research biologists had not really broached the idea that toxins ingested by a woman could cause cancer in her fetus. Toxins were thought either to kill or malform outright; resistance ran strong to the thought that somewhere between death and teratogenesis there existed a dark, middle ground where toxins could initiate cell changes that would, months, years, or even decades later, proclaim themselves as cancer in the person that the fetus had become.

This resistance is somewhat curious to explain. As early as 1947, it was known that injecting female mice with certain highly reactive agents could result in cancers of the lung among their offspring, and in the 1960s, tumors of the nervous system and the trachea were added to the list of prenatally induced cancers. These experiments, however, were not considered a warning for the human condition. Perhaps biological scientists, just subconsciously, avoided the idea of people's being destined to the most dreaded of diseases even before birth—although the sardonic comment of one cancer specialist is that "these are just the sort of grim things which interest us most." Perhaps medical scientists, not unlike the French with their dreamy faith in the Maginot line, were simply accustomed to believing that this was one disaster against which the placental barrier would hold firm. In any case, the scattered animal work with transplacental carcinogens was mostly ignored until 1971. That year, biologists and cancer specialists from around the world hastily convened in Hanover, West Germany, for the first international conference on transplacental carcinogenesis, breathless to try to determine what humankind had to deal with now.

By the 1950s, cancer had already become the largest disease killer of children under fifteen in many industrial nations, and it was tempting, at first, to think that transplacental carcinogenesis would explain cancers that skipped their usual latency period to claim the health of babies and young children. But the animal work to date points toward a far different conclusion. Carcinogenic exposures in early life appear, above all, to be latent contributors to the runaway incidence of *adult* cancers. "What we have seen with overwhelming predominance in rodents," comments Jerry Rice, the artful scientist who is head of the Perinatal Carcinogenesis Section at the National Cancer Institute, "is that the types of transplacentally induced tumors which develop tend to be associated with adult life and even old age in man."

It is instructive, against this background of malignant delay, to consider the general bearing of transplacental and juvenile exposures on the steady rise of adult cancer rates now common in the industrialized world. In 1900, only 3.9 percent of all deaths in the United States were the work of cancer; by 1970, 17.2 percent of all American deaths were attributable to this cause, and the increase was not just because more people now live to an age when cancer "naturally" develops; about half this increase is considered to represent new cases that would never have occurred at the turn of the century, even had the lifespan been equal. One can, of course, never repeat too often that people have brought a lot of this trouble on themselves through smoking—and drinking. While alcohol does not seem to be an outright carcinogen, it does enhance the carcinogenicity of cigarettes. Some cancer specialists now think that about 30 percent of male cancer deaths are the combined work of cigarettes and liquor.

That said, there has still been a great increase in other cancers. And the circumstances of the increase hold a promise that cancer rates will accelerate even faster in the future. It is crucial to realize that most patients dying from cancer today are people whose youthful and prenatal exposure to toxins was a fraction of those being sustained by children today. In 1900, for example, there was no such thing as a synthetic organic pesticide. DDT, the first one, was synthesized in 1939; by 1970, almost one billion pounds of "pesticidal active ingredients" were being sold annually in the United States. In 1900, about the only synthetic food additives were the coal-tar colors; by the 1970s, the average annual consumption of synthetic food chemicals had reached about two pounds per person. In 1900, there could hardly have been said to be a chemical industry: by the 1970s, chemists were synthesizing some 6,000 new substances a week—arrangements of atoms never before existent on the earth.

In 1900, there was one asbestos mine in all of North America—an enterprise in Quebec; from World War II to the present, some eight to eleven million Americans have sustained workplace exposures to asbestos. In 1976, in preliminary tracing of the families of the workers at just one factory, the Environmental Health Laboratory at Mt. Sinai Laboratory in New York uncovered four cases of pleural mesothelioma among the now middle-aged children of one-time asbestos workers. Pleural mesothelioma is a characteristic and invariably fatal chest cancer, which often follows asbestos exposure. Apparently these children had been condemned to develop it, thirty or forty years previously, by breathing the asbestos dust and fibers brought home on their parents' workclothes. (That same year, Dr. Irving Selikoff, the head of the Environmental Health Laboratory, revealed that thousands of pounds of modeling clay ordered for New York City schools contained up to 50 percent asbestos; its particular combination of malleability and indestructibility—in the happy jargon of industrial public relations, asbestos is known as "the magic mineral"—had made asbestos a favored ingredient for endless consumer products, from brake linings to insulation material.)

That asbestos, like DES, causes a characteristic cancer has permitted some confirmation of its latent malignancy. Whether some of these other substances, food additives, "pesticidal active ingredients," and new chemicals are causing or will cause later cancer in people who encountered them as children is not fully known. It is hard not to wonder, however, what the American cancer rate will be when infants birthed to the present deluge take their own turn as adults.

DES, in dramatizing the importance of early exposures to toxins, opened a startling new vista into cancer causation and prospects; it also opened a new vista into the very nature of carcinogens. Without the impetus of their cancer, probably no one would have thought to monitor the DES children. With the impetus of cancer, they have become one of the most closely watched populations in the world. Cancer is not their sole problem. Suspected or confirmed problems with the DES children now range from diminished fertility to subtle alterations in personality; they have provided the graphic human example of something already evident from animal research—that when a carcinogen does reach the fetus, cancer may just be the obvious signpost that other cells or tissues were injured in various ways.

The exposé of stilbestrol (DES) began in the spring of 1966. Dr. Howard Ulfelder, a courtly, blue-eyed physician who was then Chief of the Gynecological Service at Massachusetts General Hospital, encountered a teenage girl with clear-cell adenocarcinoma of the vagina that spring—the first such case in his medical experience. A glandular cancer, clear-cell adenocarcinoma is usually found in women over age fifty. It is so rare in the young that, at the time, the known cases among women under age thirty recorded in the entire world medical literature totaled precisely three. But cancer, that strange expression of cells gone wild with life and multiplying without boundaries, endlessly assumes rare forms and unexpected twists. This first case, referred to him by a colleague, did not elicit much worry until the next year, when Dr. Ulfelder encountered two more teenage patients with the same disease. "My nurse says I just came out of the examining room shaking my head," he recalls. "Clearly this was more than coincidence. We questioned these patients intensely about possible factors, but we were not really sure what we were after, or how to find it. Then, one day, the mother of the second patient said to me, 'You know, doctor, you've asked me a lot of questions about this girl, but there's one thing I just remembered. When I was pregnant, I was given DES to prevent miscarriage. Do you suppose that had a connection with this tumor?"

"I don't see how it could," was Ulfelder's immediate reply.

From the perspective of decades, it is hard to appreciate the remarkable faith DES once enjoyed. Its synthesis in 1938 by Sir Charles Dodds presented the world with the first synthetic estrogen and generated an exciting, heady promise that all sorts of biological secrets were on the point of being mastered. What generated supreme confidence in DES use during pregnancy was that its major advocates as a "support" were a golden couple of American medical science—Dr. George Van Siclen Smith, from 1942 to 1967 the head of the Gynecology Department at Harvard Medical School, and Dr. Olive Watkins Smith, a Radcliffe graduate and biochemist. The Smiths had married in 1930 and plunged into what would become their lifelong work of researching reproduction and hormones. In the early 1940s, they began prescribing DES to women with a poor pregnancy prognosis—for example, diabetic women, and women with a history of miscarriage. After what appeared to be an initial success with troubled pregnancies, they went on to prescribe DES randomly for several hundred other pregnancies, variously reporting back in the *American Journal of Obstetrics and Gynecology* that infants born to DES mothers were "bigger," "healthier," and "more rugged" than other children.

Looking back over these yellowing reports of seemingly healthy children being delivered to woman after woman with a previous history of miscarriage, it is easy to see how the Smiths, and other people, became entranced. The Smiths' early success may have been random luck; or, through enthusiasm alone, they may have helped many tense, fearful women, expecting another miscarriage and more disappointment, to make it through a pregnancy. A comparison of pregnancy outcome among normal mothers given DES and untreated normal mothers also looked promising; the DES mothers had fewer stillbirths and their babies weighed more at birth. But there was a hint of trouble: given in high doses before the twentieth week, DES itself was associated with a high risk of miscarriage. There was also a snare: the Smiths had not compared the DES women on a regimen of placebo tablets—a research technique that eliminates psychological bias. In 1953, a research group at the University of Chicago that did compare DES women with placebo women found no advantage in pregnancy outcome with the use of the hormone. Stilbestrol's carcinogenicity to animals, moreover, was well documented within a few years of its synthesis. At one point, even Sir Charles Dodds had inveighed against the use of synthetic estrogen as a pregnancy support.

In the heady atmosphere of the times, none of this caused much second thought—or, at least people with second thoughts kept them quietly to themselves. To its believers, DES was a sort of Sputnik of baby production, a substance that could build bigger, better, bouncier human beings. Because Boston had been the center for the first human trials of the drug, in the end it became the center for the first outbreak of DES cancers.

"Well," comments Dr. Ulfelder, "at least that second mother had given us a clue. When the next case turned up, I asked the mother about DES and she, too, had used it."

In 1971, Dr. Ulfelder and his colleagues, Dr. Arthur Herbst and Dr. David Poskanzer, put together the preliminary findings about DES in an article in the *New England Journal of Medicine*. Titled "Adenocarcinoma of the Vagina: Association of Maternal Stilbestrol Therapy with Tumor Appearance in Young Women," it reported on the then eight known cases of DES cancer; and it probably caused as much medical panic as has any such report. The form of cancer was fatal in about 15 percent of cases—a figure that may come down as these young women learn to seek early examination—and it often condemned young women to surgery that precluded their ever having children. The real worry, however, was that millions of pregnant women had taken the stuff. Medical scientists shuddered to the same thought that had struck Dr. Ulfelder. "I imagined," he remembers, "that this was just the tip of the iceberg here. I could visualize our going into the late 1970s with thousands of cases."

On that thought began one of the stranger medical and social odysseys in contemporary history. What do you do when you know that up to six million people—mothers and their daughters and sons—have been exposed to a particularly powerful carcinogen? For millions of people, physicians, patients, and public alike, DES has now brought home the reality of headlines and cancer scares that once seemed remote; it is the tragedy that landed on their doorsteps with the morning paper.

The problem in estimating the risk for genital cancers in DES women concerns changes in the genital tract caused by the drug. These changes are largely focused on the junction of the cervix and vagina. Two important tissues—the squamous tissue lining the vagina and the glandular and cystic structures along the cervical wall, which are known as columnar epithelium—meet as this junction. Officially termed the squamo-columnar junction, but known in the slang of gynecology as "where the action is," it is where cervical cancer invariably originates even in normal circumstances. It seems that, like nervous soldiers guarding a disputed border, this meeting of diverse tissues just contains an unusual malignant potential. In normal women, the junction—and "the field of action"—is confined to 4 centimeters or so. DES, however, usually causes the columnar epithelium to creep some centimeters out of the cervical opening and often causes separate patches of this tissue to form on the vaginal wall. DES women, as it is often put, have "a normal tissue in an abnormal place." In its abnormal placement, the tissue becomes known as adenosis.

In theory, this adenosis, all of it surrounded by "little squamo-columnar junctions" expands the area of risk, perhaps ten-, twenty-, thirty-fold or more, depending on an individual woman's condition. In practice, it is questionable whether the DES-inspired adenosis patches in the vagina embody the same malignant potential as a natural squamo-columnar junction. The vagina has actually proven the preferred location for DES cancers (the ratio of vaginal to cervical tumors is running about two to one), but the form of the cancer that has developed in DES daughters, clear-cell adeno-carcinoma, is among the rarest cancers known. The usual cancer that develops at the junction is a squamous-type cancer; and it usually appears after age thirty-five.

Some physicians had at first feared that the real trouble for DES daughters would begin when they reached the age for squamous tumors. Dr. Adolf Stafl, Assistant Professor of Obstetrics at the Medical College of Wisconsin, for one, has felt almost from the first discovery of the problems with DES—and still feels—that perhaps "the major clinical risk for DES-exposed girls is the future development of squamous neoplasia." The only reason Dr. Stafl sees to modify this position is that DES daughters do not seem to engage in either early or very active sex lives (pursuits that, for reasons that remain obscure, predispose women toward later cervical cancer). Their internal embarrassment often keeps them away from men and from sex. "So I would say that's the only thing that changes the situation at all," comments Stafl. Other observers, however, are more encouraged. With time, the extra adenosis patches in many young women appear to be healing or receding of their own accord, and pathologists are generally not finding an unusual amount of "precancerous" squamous tissue in the genital tracts of these young women. Only time, however, can provide the final answer about squamous cancers. Most DES daughters are not yet even thirty years old.

The irony is that adenocarcinoma, the cancer that first launched the DES scare, has not turned out to be a major risk. It has a striking age pattern, with most victims being between the ages of fourteen and twenty-two, and a huge peak in cases at age nineteen. Dr. Herbst, now Chairman of Obstetrics-Gynecology at the University of Chicago Pritzker School of Medicine, believes this pattern suggests that "DES probably isn't a complete carcinogen and that other factors are involved in carcinogenesis. It appears some of them are associated with the onset of puberty." In any case, by 1977, only 333 total cases of suspected transplacental genital cancers in young women had been reported to the DES Registry—or, as it is officially known, the Registry for Research on Hormonal Transplacental Carcinogenesis—being jointly maintained by the University of Chicago and Massachusetts General Hospital. Meanwhile, thousands of young women had passed through adolescence cancer-free. Based on their experience, Dr. Herbst, in well-accepted figures, has projected that the ultimate adenocarcinoma cases will probably be limited to between one in 1000 and one in 10,000 DES daughters.

These figures, however, apply only to DES. Natural progesterone, derived from animals, was also used as a pregnancy support, as were synthetic progestins, natural estrogen, and even testosterone, the male hormone. Three cases of adenocarcinoma have now been reported to the DES Registry in which natural progesterone alone was the agent the mother had taken. It is still too early to know whether these progesterone cases signal a trend and whether more thousands of mothers, daughters, and sons are at risk. There has been no official advice or pronouncements, like those for DES, on progesterone or other types of supports. "We are simply trying to work our way through DES," says a member of the DES Task Force. "Progesterone has not come up yet."

Much can be learned about DES because there is an almost perfect control population against which the DES group can be compared. In the early 1950s, the late Dr. W. J. Dieckmann, of the University of Chicago Department of Obstetrics and Gynecology, decided to run a major trial comparing pregnancy outcome among women given DES and a carefully matched population given a placebo. The Dieckmann group found "no differences in the strength, vigor, nursing ability, weight . . . and other criteria of growth and development in babies born of mothers who received stilbestrol and those who had taken placebos." And the DES group actually experienced somewhat higher rates of miscarriages and neonatal deaths. Dr. Dieckmann concluded that DES was of no value in pregnancy—as did two somewhat similar studies done almost simultaneously.

Unfortunately, even when published in the *American Journal of Obstetrics and Gynecology,* the Chicago results did not quell the breathless enthusiasm for DES. The *Journal* itself continued to print as many full-page ads as drug companies cared to purchase promoting DES as "assurance of a successful pregnancy." More unfortunately, in keeping with the paltry ethics of the time, the University of Chicago had not bothered to tell the DES women they were part of an experiment, or even what drug they were taking. The University has paid for this lapse in several million dollars' worth of legal suits. The one benefit of the Chicago study seems to have been retrospective; there now exists a defined DES population and a control group that can provide considerable insight into the problems awaiting thousands of other mothers and children and the attention they require.

These insights suggest that the DES drama has a long time yet to play. A few years ago, a nurse at the University of Chicago, who was taking health histories of the DES daughters, was struck by the number of their mothers—the women who originally took the drug—who seemed to have died of breast cancer. The University of Chicago then started studying cancer cases among the mothers. In 1977, by litigating under the Freedom of Information Act, Public Citizen, the Ralph Nader group, made public a preliminary report on the situation which the university had filed with the National Institutes of Health. DES mothers, at that time, had twice the breast cancer incidence and triple the breast cancer deaths of control mothers. Moreover, their breast cancers were appearing at an earlier age.

In 1978, after completing a twenty-five-year follow-up of more than 1200 DES mothers and controls, the University of Chicago confirmed that the DES women did have more than double the overall cancer deaths, and it confirmed that their fatal malignancies were mainly breast cancers. The university, however, in an interpretation of its own figures which many observers regard as "nothing short of absolute nonsense," considers that the mothers' cancer rate still lies within the bounds of chance. The Mayo Clinic has not found a breast cancer excess among its own population of DES mothers, but, again, that is not cause for much comfort. The doses given to mothers at the Mayo Clinic were far below those administered at the University of Chicago. In late 1978, the DES Task Force, an advisory group formed by the Department of Health, Education and Welfare, officially commented that, while a breast cancer excess among DES mothers was "not established," it found "cause for serious concern over the drug's carcinogenic potential in this population." The Task Force also sternly advised DES mothers, especially those under age fifty, against responding to this concern by having routine mammograms, or breast X rays. Experimental work has now shown that estrogen and radiation may enhance each other's potential to cause breast tumors.

Another problem possibly awaiting the DES daughters concerns reproductive potential. As of 1976, almost 20 percent of those DES daughters who had been found and questioned were experiencing irregular menstruation—almost double the rate of menstrual difficulties seen among the control daughters. Almost double the control daughters, meanwhile, had been pregnant. Evidently both conceiving and carrying children to term will be difficult for some of these young women.

Investigating the reproductive health of DES children also brought into focus something often overlooked—namely that half the DES babies were boys. They may be destined for even more serious reproductive problems than the girls. About one quarter of the sons traced by the University of Chicago have various genital abnormalities. Most of these are benign cysts, but others, including microphallus and undescended testes, are both psychologically and medically important. Microphallus, of course, is a permanent condition. Undescended testes, while often easy to correct with surgery, also predisposes to testicular cancer.

The real questions about the reproductive future of DES sons, however, has come from examining their sperm. In theory, of course, only one sperm is needed to make a baby; but in practice, a sperm count below 20 million per milliliter of semen raises some doubt of conception and a count below 10 million raises considerable doubt. One quarter of the DES sons, but not one son in the control population, tested below 20 million. Sperm shape is a second important measure of sperm quality. Although it has not been conclusively proven that abnormally shaped sperm represent mutations, biologists now believe that mutation is the main reason sperm assume strange, unwieldy shapes. Since normal sperm are adept at reaching the egg first, the small proportion of abnormal shapes found in the semen of virtually all men is not a focus of much worry. As, however, the proportion of abnormal sperm rises, so does the chance that one of their number will manage to reach and fertilize an egg. In the DES sons, this proportion is great indeed. One quarter of them had 40 percent or more abnormal shapes—a sperm debacle, again, not evident in any son among the controls. Hundreds of DES sons, as are hundreds of DES daughters, are already parents to healthy children; but others clearly are not going to be able to father a child. "They have different reactions to this," comments Dr. William Gill, a University of Chicago urologist who has worked closely with the DES sons. "In the beginning, some just acted pretty macho and said they never wanted children anyway. But, as they get a little older, we're beginning to get complaints. Still, it's too early to tell the real extent of infertility."

Almost everyone dealing with the aftermath of DES is aware of another question about the sons' future—a question that, however, goes mostly unmentioned in medical journals, HEW reports, and conference discussions. There is substantial animal evidence that hormone manipulation at critical points of prenatal development can alter normal sexual orientation. Comparing sexual behavior between animals and man is, of course, hardly the same as comparing cancer cells or kidney damage. Human sexuality involves conditioning, love, psychological interludes, and, for that matter, physical positions that have no counterpart in rat sex. No research group has yet tried to quantify the sexual impact of

DES on humans; and perhaps no research group ever will. The "perfect" population at Chicago may be the sole scientifically valid population in the country from which to determine whether prenatal exposure to this "female" hormone has, even if occasionally, caused men to be homosexual. There are doctors and researchers at Chicago willing to do the epidemiology; but the university is not willing to have it done. Although it has been more ethical than many other institutions—and private physicians—in monitoring its DES population, the university does not care to invite more explosives by broaching the subject of homosexuality.

The DES children, however—and not just those at Chicago, but the other hundreds of thousands of them—have at least the right to obtain as clear an idea as possible of what did or did not happen to them. They should not have to stand alone, wondering about themselves.

The progression of discovery for DES daughters was to go from cancer to "lesser" concerns about their reproductive potential. The progression for DES sons has been the opposite. In 1978, a few years after the University of Chicago first reported on the sons' genital abnormalities and "pathological sperm," the Memorial Sloan-Kettering Cancer Institute in New York reported that 10 percent of almost 150 testicular cancer cases referred there in recent years had occurred in young men with a documented DES exposure—and other cases involved suspected DES exposure. Not one of the young men in a control group with other cancers had been exposed to DES.

Although many commentators, including the DES Task Force, still refer to the Sloan-Kettering findings as "preliminary," it would be more surprising if DES didn't cause testicular cancer. The Sloan-Kettering findings stand out against both the known malignant potential of undescended testes and against a doubling of testicular cancer cases among white males—and a tripling of cases among black males—since 1950. Because some increase in testicular cancer has been seen in countries where DES was never used as a pregnancy support, or as an additive to the feed of beef and poultry—a use permitted in the United States through July 1979—the hormone is not the sole agent under suspicion in the testicular cancer increase. Clearly, however, there is a high risk for the DES sons. Some people now recommend that, at least, they be coached to examine themselves for external lumps that may be a warning of malignancy. Treatment of testicular cancer involves castration of the affected testicle always, chemotherapy usually, and radiation treatment sometimes. The five-year survival rate for men who were treated in the mid-1960s has proven to be about 70 percent, and treatment advances since then are thought to have brought the figure higher.

Usually it is impossible to trace ordinary cancers to a single cause some ten, twenty, or thirty years after induction. Not all cancers, of course, are caused by environmental agents; but those that are become hopelessly lost in the mass of cancers. They are not "distinguishable" from non-environmental cancers; their cells do not wear little signs calling attention to their origin.

Since cancer causes cannot be traced, in effect, no real cost-benefit accounting is possible for suspicious consumer products. The food and drug industries, not to mention other industries, complain a lot about the costs of pretesting their products. Although the drug industry has now, for years, engaged in some pretesting, the rest of the industrial world was able to excuse itself from that obligation until 1976. In that year, Congress finally passed the Toxic Substances Control Act, a piece of legislation that, if basically hedging, may see chemical products more thoroughly studied before they enter the marketplace. To animal-test a new product for carcinogenicity costs about $200,000—a figure that rapid-assay systems like the Ames test are already bringing down and will eventually bring down further. Since a fatal case of cancer may now easily consume $20,000 in medical care, even a "mild" carcinogen, which caused very few cancers, would obviously lose ground fast in any real accounting of costs and benefits. But DES is the great exception in cost accounting; because the rare adenocarcinomas can be traced, its bill has fallen due.

To statisticians, the small number of DES cancer cases to date may be reassuring; to families living in the "psychological reality" Laurie Sale has described, these numbers have little meaning. It is not in the nature of mothers to sit and watch their own children become fatal, if rare, cancer cases; and DES children old enough to understand their own situation are no more inclined to just let statistics take their impersonal course. The only obvious way to try to keep DES children from premature death is an extensive program of attention and monitoring, which may well last as long as they live, and which, because they can be internally examined, has largely focused on the daughters.

The National Cancer Institute has recommended that all DES daughters receive "a thorough pelvic examination at menarche or if they have reached fourteen years of age. Younger girls should be examined if they develop abnormal bleeding or discharge." The costs of DES begin with the complex and exhausting medical effort required by this recommendation. The first step has been just to alert people to their possible danger. Many women prescribed stilbestrol may not have even known for sure what it was. (A lot of them seemed to think they were taking vitamins.) In 1978, New York State launched a $300,000 program that may serve as the general model for carrying out the National Cancer Institute recommendation. These funds are being used both to set up screening centers around the state and to underwrite a media campaign to tell young women to be examined.

What to do after the initial examination is still under debate. In the beginning, there was a rush to remove the adenosis patches. (Actually, the first panic also saw a few girls subjected to unnecessary vaginectomies.) Although a minority of physicians still insist on removing adenosis patches, most physicians now leave the patches alone, except when they cause a discomforting discharge, and simply examine the DES daughters once or twice yearly.

For most of the DES daughters, these examinations will be

physically uneventful, but a few young women may be found to have "premalignant" tissue changes known as dysplasia and carcinoma in situ. As is adenosis, dysplasia is a subject for some disagreement. Since it usually does not advance to cancer, some physicians also incline toward leaving dysplasia alone; others remove it. Carcinoma in situ is an unquestioned candidate for removal, but doctors can still work up a quite heated argument over the proper method of removal. Extensive carcinoma in situ calls for surgery; but small patches are candidates for localized techniques such as cryosurgery (freezing) and lasers. In a recent *Medical World News* roundup on the subject, a laser advocate huffily termed cryosurgery "wanting" and a doctor who preferred cryosurgery described the laser as "just expensive cautery." There are, however, no arguments over the response to outright cancer. The response is a radical vaginectomy. Since the operation involves removing the vagina, cervix, and uterus, it precludes future pregnancy; the vagina, however, is reconstructed to allow the woman to have intercourse.

In a sense, the initial physical examinations may be the most difficult step for DES daughters—but not because they are painful. Except for the sting of an iodine smear used to confirm the presence of adenosis, or a brief twinge should a physician take a "biopsy bite" of genital tissue for laboratory analysis, these examinations are not a painful experience. They do, however, seem to be a jolting way for young girls to first encounter their own bodies. Like many people, Fran Fishbane—a DES mother from Long Island and a co-founder of DES Action, a nationwide organization of families—has begun to think that "the emotional damage to the DES-exposed and their families is far more significant than the medical." In counseling the children, she often finds that the daughters think of themselves as "freaks." They fantasize about "odors of decay" coming from their bodies, and tend to think that sex is permanently forbidden to them "because a guy could catch cancer from me." And, in counseling the parents, she finds a common thread of emotional exhaustion and malaise. The mothers are often plunged into relentless guilt; the fathers are worried, confused, but fatherishly inarticulate.

An essential hurdle is to prepare the daughters properly for their first exam. Laurie Sale, in a technique many mothers have adopted, has taken her daughter along on her own gynecological examinations since the child was seven. The idea is to instill in her that this is not something to fear and that "Mommy does this for her own health, too." The DES groups are finding, however, that physicians may need as much preparation as these young patients. The difference between dealing with grown women and dealing with preteenagers seems to be little understood among gynecologists. Fran Fishbane was stunned by an instructional film, shown at a DES conference she attended, that was meant to guide doctors in the psychology of handling very young and very nervous patients. The film showed an eleven-year-old girl being brought in for her first exam. She was crying and visibly trembling. "The presiding doctor just remarked that this is the kind of behavior you have to put up with all the time," she recalls. "And he said not to pay attention and just get on with the exam."

A particular complaint is that some gynecologists insist on surgically disposing of the hymen of younger patients. Although surgical dehymenization is a minor surgical procedure, hardly requiring a few snips of the scissors, it is hard to imagine many simple actions that could be more psychologically explosive. Parents have reported that it brings out specific fears that "sex is like that" and often leaves behind a shaken child. Taking all these factors together, Fran Fishbane has commented that she remains "gloomy about the DES child going for her first exam. Almost without exception, she goes ill-prepared, burdened by her mother's anxiety and guilt. I can envision a future of emotional celibates on a collective analytic couch, all equating their first DES exam with medical and emotional rape."

On the other hand, those physicians who have really strained to think about this special population have found ways to soothe and reassure them. One person who has thought hard is Dr. Norma Perez-Veridiano, a slight, smiling woman who heads the DES Screening Clinic at Brookdale Hospital in Brooklyn, New York. Dr. Veridiano's first idea is that the very young DES daughters should not even be examined internally on the first visit.

She has found that "they are usually so petrified already that scaring them more means you may lose them forever. They simply refuse to come back." Instead, Dr. Veridiano employs the first visit to just take a history and look over the children externally, actions that seem to reassure them into returning. Dr. Veridiano has also made it something of a personal quest to seek out small instruments adapted to the younger girls. With them, for example, she substitutes a nasal speculum, an instrument usually used to hold open the nose for examination, for the standard gynecological speculum. She has examined children as young as seven without once having had to remove a hymen surgically. These may be less than pleasant details about the aftermath of DES; but they are the details people find themselves having to think about. A new use for nasal speculums is part of the cost accounting.

It is perhaps a measure of its emotional impact that not even physicians are immune to the particular strain of DES. For physicians, part of the problem is that they are dealing with what they know to be a medically caused disease. But part of the problem for them, like everyone else, is that the DES population is young and that their sex organs are the main target of damage, an idea that seems to invoke other people's sense of vulnerability as would no other target. From the waiting rooms of clinics where mothers sit in grim expectation while a daughter is examined, to the cluttered hospital offices where the statisticians put together new numbers, the whole subject has an edge of weariness, not to say exhaustion. Dr. Marluce Bibbo, the chief investigator of the first Chicago study of DES sons, remembers the tightness in her stomach many nights when she went home. "Now sometimes when we call up," she says in the lilting accents of her native Brazil, "they tell us just to leave them out of the study. They don't want to be reminded anymore. They don't want to know anything else about it." "I don't care what kind of personality you have, how strong a doctor you are," Dr. Veridiano says in the soft accents of her native Philippines, "seeing a nineteen-year-old with cancer gets to you."

It is hard to see how, in the end, anyone escapes a tragedy of the dimension of DES. The 250,000 to three million women who took it, their affected children, and their other immediate family members form a not-insignificant portion of the American population for whom this worry is now an irrevocable part of life. The financial cost for examining DES daughters for the first time and for keeping a medical watch on both the sons and daughters over the years will be staggering. And, whether ostensibly paid by government programs, insurance companies, lawsuit settlements, or the families themselves, these costs will, to some degree, be borne by everyone. Maybe, after all, it is the final lesson of DES that no one truly escapes; it has reverberated everywhere, sending parents to pacing hospital corridors, sending physicians home feeling sick to their stomachs, sending copywriters to devising media campaigns of advice and warning, and sending young women to vent their rage at group sessions formed for mutual support.

The drug industry, however, is not weary.

In May 1977, the *Wall Street Journal* reported that the legal suits filed against present and former manufacturers of DES then totaled more than $3.5 billion. Yet DES remains very cheap to produce—and it remains in wide distribution in the United States and elsewhere. The *Wall Street Journal* has also reported that, as late as 1974, American doctors wrote some 11,000 prescriptions for DES to be used during pregnancy. While it is hard to imagine under what sandpile the prescribing physicians had their heads buried, it is true the FDA had taken little action against DES at that time. Governments elsewhere were even slower to move. On a trip through South America in 1976, Fran Fishbane observed DES still being given to unsuspecting pregnant women in Argentina, Costa Rica, Brazil, and Venezuela. It is nothing new, however, that drugs disapproved in the Western world remain on sale in less-developed countries. A Swedish manufacturer of thalidomide kept that teratogen on the market in Argentina for three months following its ban on home ground.

In the United States, synthetic estrogen retains FDA approval for several purposes and seems, in any case, to have become one of those drugs now so integrated into medical practice that FDA statements about its "appropriate" uses are not much heeded. The Health Research Group has managed to make public the number of DES prescriptions, and their uses, for the year ending June 1977. During that time, American doctors wrote 121,000 DES prescriptions for the purpose of relieving breast engorgement or to suppress lactation following the delivery of a child. They prescribed DES and other estrogens 3000 times as a treatment for acne, a use not approved by the FDA. And they prescribed estrogens in general 59,000 times—and DES in particular 3000 times—for "prophylaxis." Since estrogens in large doses may prevent the implantation of a fertilized egg, this prescription explanation presumably means the estrogen was used as a "morning-after contraceptive." The FDA only approves estrogens as morning-after contraceptives in instances of rape or incest; the 59,000 figure suggests that physicians have not limited their prescribing to these two situations.

A few years ago, the Health Research Group requested the FDA to restrict the availability of DES as a morning-after contraceptive by categorizing it as "an investigational new drug." The FDA has declined to place DES in this restricted category, but, in 1978, the agency did order an end to the marketing of the huge 25-milligram tablets (they contain about the estrogen dose of a two-years' supply of birth control pills) used for "morning-after" purposes. The agency has also begun the necessary formal process to withdraw its approval of prescribing DES as a lactation suppressant—a move virtually mandated by the confirmation of breast cancer in the Chicago DES mothers. (It seems only fair to point out that the current administration of the FDA is burdened by a huge backload of inaction from previous administrations. Since DES was a proven animal carcinogen by 1940 and has been a proven human carcinogen since 1971, restrictive actions should have come years, if not decades, ago.) Meanwhile, Fran Fishbane reports that at least forty baby girls, born since 1977 and exposed to DES when their mothers were given it as a morning-after pill, have come to her group's attention. Either DES failed to prevent implantation or the women, without realizing it, were already quite pregnant.

*

The focus on DES as a pregnancy support has somewhat deflected concern about its use as a feed additive. In 1947, poultry producers began dosing their birds with DES to make them gain weight faster. In 1954 the cattle industry followed suit by adding DES to the feed of its animals. Since then, DES has been a steady, if very low-level, component of the American diet. Whether or not residues of DES in meat could cause cancer is "something," comments Dr. Robert Scully, the Massachusetts General pathologist who has worked on DES from the beginning, "that I don't think anyone could say with certainty. We just don't know the smallest possible dose which could be cancer-causing." The use of DES as an animal feed does, however, stand out against a striking fact: for one quarter of the youthful adenocarcinoma cases reported to the DES Registry, there is no record or memory of the mother's having taken *any* special medicine during the pregnancy—whether or not she knew it to be DES. Some women, of course, may well have forgotten about medicines taken ten, twenty, or thirty years in the past; but women tend to have a very high recall for "special treatments" or occurrences during pregnancy and, in any case, maternal memories about DES have often been cross-checked against available hospital and physician records and even by searching out other places of record—say, a local drugstore—where a dusty stilbestrol prescription might yet be on file. If there is no way to creditably prove that some of these cases represent cancers caused by DES in food, there are credible reasons to think it possible they could.

One reason is the huge residues that were common in the

early years when there was no control over DES use in animals. Poultry producers, for example, simply began to implant pellets of the stuff directly in the necks of chickens—a practice that seems to have inspired the first DES lawsuit. In the early 1950s, mink ranchers went to court when their animals became sterile after being fed the heads and necks of DES-treated chickens. Testing at about that time revealed that the skin fat of treated chickens commonly contained about 20 to 30 parts per billion of DES—far above the dosage required to cause breast cancer in mice. In 1959, in one of the few outright acts of indignation in its history, the FDA suspended all DES use in poultry, a suspension that remains in effect. In 1971, the FDA mandated that all estrogen feeding of cattle must be stopped a week before slaughter. Presumably, this would be time enough to allow the DES to fully clear the animals' bodies. In actual fact, DES residues are still constantly found in beef. In late 1975, Dr. Sydney Wolfe complained that sampling had shown residue "levels as high as 11 parts per billion . . . an increase from levels found in meat sampled earlier in 1975." In 1977, sampling of cattle livers, the organ where DES tends to concentrate, turned up residues in more than 1 percent of samples tested. The Department of Agriculture, by the way, samples so few cattle—1454 beef livers were tested for DES in 1977—that it is hard to know whether these numbers represent the general exposure to DES. A little carelessness by a few ranchers could, without anyone's knowing it, subject thousands of people to higher residues and, to judge from animal experiments, a little carelessness with DES might go quite a long way. Merely adding 6.5 ppb to the daily diet of mice causes a large incidence of breast cancer among the female animals. In 1975 hearings before the Senate Health Subcommittee, Dr. Frank Rauscher, then head of the National Cancer Institute, was asked whether pregnant women should consume meat containing any estrogen residues whatsoever. He replied with two words: "Certainly not."

Its simple potency, then, is one thing that speaks of the danger of DES residue in food. Another is the odd cancer ratio of young women in the DES Registry who are not believed to have been exposed to hormone supports; they have a ratio of vaginal to cervical tumors of about one to two—"quite the reverse," in Dr. Ulfelder's term, of the two-to-one vaginal to cervical ratio seen among women whose mothers were known to have taken DES while pregnant. Before the first reports of DES cancers, the world medical literature contained only three reported cases of vaginal adenocarcinomas in women under age thirty, compared with about thirty to sixty reports of cervical adenocarcinomas in this age group. (It is sometimes hard to judge the age of the women in older reports.) These figures suggest that the "natural" vaginal to cervical ratio for adenocarcinomas in young women runs at about one to ten or twenty.

Do these different ratios say anything about the cause of the tumors in the different groups? Dr. Ulfelder's view is that the reason the known DES group has a high ratio of vaginal tumors is simply that synthetic estrogen preferentially struck at the vagina. "If you look at how few vaginal adenocarcinomas there were before DES," he adds, "you could almost say that adenocarcinoma of the vagina was created by DES." However, even before DES, Ulfelder points out, one or two cases a year of evidently spontaneous adenocarcinoma of the cervix were turning up in young women. Since physicians have now been alerted to report all their genital cancer cases in young women to the DES Registry, the "unknown" group in the registry, with its heavy predominance of cervical tumors, probably contains the several natural cases that would have occurred during these years in any case.

Dr. Ulfelder's explanation commands perfect logic. Still, looking at the way the vaginal-to-cervical ratio of the "unknown" group falls right between the ratio of documented DES cases and the "natural" ratio, it is hard to suppress a question: were DES residues in cattle and poultry just enough to cause some adenocarcinomas without sustaining the emphatic change in ratio seen in those young women exposed to the higher doses in medication?

Americans who fret over the contents of their food supply know that the Delaney Amendment outrightly forbids the addition to foods of chemicals that cause cancer in animals—much less chemicals already proven to cause cancer in humans. The Delaney Amendment is one of the few pieces of clear, unequivocal legislation that a lobbyist-dominated Congress has ever put in the hands of an often confused and beleaguered FDA. But, in the case of DES, this most spectacular carcinogen, Congress saw fit to retract the Delaney Amendment. In 1962, it exempted DES, and some other known carcinogenic feed additives—also still in use— from the Delaney Amendment under the condition that they be employed in a way that left no residues. At the time, the crude equipment available for routine testing could not pick up small traces of DES. In 1971, however, when routine testing down to 2 ppb became possible, it also became evident that people had consistently been consuming DES residues all along. The next year, the FDA "revoked approval" of DES as an additive to animal feed. The meat industry not only managed to block this revocation in court, it also managed to block a ban on DES that Congress itself finally passed in 1975. Only in mid-1979 was the FDA finally able to invoke a DES ban that apparently will be final; and even with DES out of the way, the US meat industry is still employing several other carcinogenic feed additives, including some hormones, that are banned in most other countries.

The exasperating aspect of DES to many people is that there is not even a nutritional benefit to offset its risks; the animal weight gained through the use of DES is mainly water and fat, not protein. In 1972, the Department of Agriculture estimated that DES in cattle was saving American consumers an average of $3.85 per capita annually. Consumers may well want to decide whether they consider this a saving worth any cancer risk—whether cancer of the vagina, breast, or testicles, and however small the risk.

✳

During the years that the DES drama has been playing on the human stage, laboratory research into carcinogens that cross the placenta has drawn a portrait of some uniquely malevolent substances. Mere teratogens deform and nothing more; thalidomide is one of these. Substances capable of transplacental carcinogenesis can act on the full spectrum of development: when encountering a fetus in the proper dose and at a crucial stage of development, a given transplacental carcinogen may also kill or maim; and, even if not an immediate cause of tumors, its effects, a World Health Organization cancer specialist comments, "may be added to the effect of similar exposures in postnatal life [and] enhance subsequent exposures to the same or other carcinogens. The embryo," he goes on, "has been found to exhibit the highest response to the carcinogenic effects of chemicals at a late stage of development and to the teratogenic effects of chemicals earlier and to the lethal earliest."

In the event, moreover, that transplacental carcinogens manage to reach the forming reproductive organs, their effects may extend to a second generation—if not even further down the line of reproduction. When pregnant rodents are injected with nitrosomethylurethane, a known carcinogen, large numbers of their offspring develop cancer as they get older. Breeding these cancer-destined male offspring with ordinary females produces ordinary pups; but breeding the cancer-destined female offspring with ordinary males produces pups who develop an excess of cancer—without, of course, ever having directly encountered the nitrosomethylurethane. The eggs from which they later developed did, however, encounter the nitrosomethylurethane when their mothers were prenatally exposed to the stuff. It is thought that some injury to the eggs at that time—perhaps "a disturbance of gene-amplification"—was the eventual cause of cancer in this generation.

Are human young, like laboratory young, vulnerable to a spectrum of effects from transplacental carcinogens? With DES, the only well-documented human transplacental carcinogen, deaths early in gestation, malformation, cancer, and mutation alike have been confirmed or strongly hinted. Only in its potential to mutate does DES somewhat differ from the available animal models. To date, in animals, it has appeared that any mutational burden from transplacental carcinogens may fall most heavily on the forming germ cells of the female; with DES, the clearest hint of mutation has come from the sons. Their large percentage of abnormally shaped sperm suggests the hormone did manage to mutate, or otherwise damage, the "stem cells" that, after sexual maturity, produce the male's constant supply of new sperm.

But, for all the recent insights into transplacental carcinogenesis, science has not discovered a means of predicting which carcinogens will be "active" and dangerous to the human fetus. In the postnatal world, where all the known human carcinogens, except arsenic, cause cancer in animals as well, there seems to be an almost universal distaste for some substances; in the prenatal world, this shared distaste falls by the wayside. The problem centers on the vagaries of the fetal enzyme system. Most carcinogens will not initiate tumors unless certain enzymes activate them. (As a hormone, DES is not typical of the great mass of enzyme-mediated carcinogens.) Toward the end of gestation, the fetus goes through an enzyme surge, which progressively increases the chance of cancer; this enzyme surge accounts for the "highest response to carcinogenic chemicals at a late stage of development." As, however, the timing of the surge differs from species to species, and even from body site to body site within a species, predicting human susceptibility to transplacental cancer from work with animals is an obscure business at best.

Transplacental carcinogenesis is not without an element of biological jest. On the one hand, its low enzyme level protects the fetus from the full assault of most carcinogens; yet, with its cells rapidly dividing, for the fetus to encounter even small amounts of an "activated" carcinogen may leave it more damaged than considerable exposure to carcinogens after birth. Something to remember here is that the human fetus is relatively more mature at birth than are common test species. Since the human maturity includes higher enzyme levels, another biological jest may be that an element of safety in transplacental carcinogenesis lies with the little mouse.

✳

Most of the substances tested in the laboratory are highly reactive agents confined to experimental uses; but some, unfortunately, are not confined anywhere. A few are common food additives and industrial compounds.

Sodium nitrite, the common meat preservative, should perhaps evoke the greatest worry about transplacental carcinogenesis of any food additive now in use. It is used to cure about 60 to 70 percent of American pork products and 10 percent of beef products. Sodium nitrite levels are particularly high in ham, bacon, bologna, hot dogs, and other "meatish" fast foods. When first added to pork in the 1920s, sodium nitrite was forthrightly known as a "color fixer" and the industry was forthrightly using it to lend a pink tinge to meat which, by age, might be entitled to a grayer hue. Nitrites, however, also protect against botulism, a rare but sometimes deadly disease. There also seems to be no very scientific idea about the levels of nitrites really needed to fight botulism. In 1978, the Department of Agriculture proposed a total ban on nitrites in baby, toddler, and junior meat foods and reduced the permissible level in cured meat from 200 parts per million to 120 ppm. The former level had been set in 1925. Looking to the future, the American government seems to be slowly but surely edging toward the action of several other countries in totally dispensing with nitrite preservatives.

Not even the meat industry, which is dead set against a nitrite ban, would argue against the evidence that these preservatives are closely allied with some of the most deadly carcinogens known. Under certain conditions, including when they are fried at high temperatures, or when they encounter several other common foods or drugs while in the stomach, nitrites form nitrosamines, a type of nitroso compound. The nitroso compounds can kill the adults of all species ever tested with them, and are also eerily efficient transplacental carcinogens. By now, several hundred mice have sacrificed their lives to pointing out that nitrosamines are great travelers; they migrate "for carcinogenesis in distant organs or for transplacental passage to the fetus with subsequent development of tumors after birth." Some nitrosamines—it is not known how many exist, or how many are actually formed from nitrites— are also teratogenic to animals.

People do, however, dispute whether these animal results have meaning for humans. The dispute has focused not on distant organs, and not on the fetus, but on a very immediate organ—the stomach. Apparently, because of peculiar local conditions, in some few parts of the world, nitrite consumption and stomach cancer do appear to be closely linked. That this link does not exist in the United States, however, has formed Exhibit A for defenders of nitrite. Richard F. Spark, an associate professor of medicine at Harvard Medical School, took up the standard theme of stomach cancer in a 1978 *New Republic* article called "Legislating Against Cancer"—the gist of which was "don't bother." "In the United States and Great Britain over the past forty years," Dr. Spark blandly pointed out, "there has been a staggering increase in [nitrite] consumption, but a striking decrease in stomach cancer." As Dr. Spark comments, the reason for the stomach cancer decrease is not known. As is evident, however, to people who have reviewed the laboratory work on nitrosamines, the rate of stomach cancer says very little about the carcinogenic activities of an agent noted for attacking "distant organs and for transplacental passage to the fetus." Whether such passage could ever be proven in humans is one thing; but not to mention it at all is another.

A second controversial additive that has given some signs of transplacental activity is the artificial sweetener saccharin. Most people are aware that early in 1977, after Canadian researchers found an excess of bladder cancer among male rats fed a 5-percent saccharin diet, the FDA proposed banning it. The saccharin level in this experiment, which was about the human equivalent of drinking 800 cans of diet soda a day, drew a lot of snickers. Congressman Andrew Jacobs of Indiana perhaps epitomized the public attitude toward the tests when he proposed that saccharin products be labeled "Warning: The Canadians have determined that saccharin is dangerous to your rat's health."

There might have been less comedy had the FDA tried to help the public understand that in a standard carcinogenicity test using fifty animals, the statistical chances of finding a cancer excess are still not that large, even when the animals are fed a fairly hefty amount of the test substance. By now, Canadian investigators have also developed preliminary—if disputed—evidence of excess bladder cancer in male humans who routinely consume saccharin products. This is not to say that saccharin is the most potent carcinogen ever tested; but it is to say it holds dangers for beings other than Canadian rats.

The Canadians immediately banned saccharin outright. The American Congress passed something called the Saccharin Study and Labeling Act. It directed that all products containing saccharin be marked with warning labels—the now-familiar admonition that "this product contains saccharin which has been determined to cause cancer in laboratory animals"—and that there be a year's study and review of the evidence against saccharin. In February 1979, the National Academy of Sciences, while "upgrading" saccharin from the classification of a "mild cancer-causing agent" to the more dangerous "moderate cancer-causing agent," did not recommend a full ban; instead, the academy favored some restrictions, especially to keep saccharin away from children. A month later, the FDA announced that it would take another year before any potential ban could go into effect.

In any case, the public information about saccharin has been so misleading that it seems doubtful the Congress, or the consuming public, would accept a ban at the present time. Because they are only familiar with the one Canadian test, most people seem to think that 800 diet sodas a day is, in fact, the danger zone for saccharin; it is, moreover, an article of faith among the public that saccharin helps reduce weight and is of great benefit to dieters and diabetics. The available evidence suggests that, to the contrary, saccharin may cause weight gains. This is because the stuff demonstrably depresses blood sugar and, when their blood sugar is low, people develop insistent cravings for food. Rodents fed saccharin, and given equal access to the food trough, gain more weight than rodents not fed this assumed weight-reducer. The Canadian Diabetes Association does not regard saccharin as being of assistance to diabetics; it supports the Canadian ban.

Many adults may nonetheless say they are willing to take saccharin with the risks, just as they do cigarettes and just as they do alcohol. It is tempting to let them have their way; saccharin would seem to be the sort of situation that Oliver Wendell Holmes had in mind when he remarked that, among their other constitutional freedoms, Americans enjoyed an unabashed right to make fools of themselves. The particular aspect of saccharin that bothers many scientists, however, is not just that saccharin products may reach children—who, of course, do not know they are making fools of themselves because they don't understand the significance of the warning labels—but that many pregnant women, in a frantic if misguided effort to curb their weight gain during pregnancy, become large consumers of the five million pounds of saccharin sold annually in the United States.

Saccharin has not only been tested on pregnant rats; it has also been tested on pregnant monkeys, bringing the results closer to the human situation. After saccharin infusion to pregnant monkeys, the sweetener clears from the maternal blood in three hours—but takes five hours to clear from the fetal blood. Autopsying these infants after their saccharin encounter has shown that the stuff made its way to all their tissues—except the central nervous system—and that even after clearing the blood, it persisted "in fetal tissue itself, frequently within the cytoplasm of individual cells." (By contrast, the previously banned artificial sweetener cyclamate does not persist in fetal tissues. For the most part, it just sloshes around in the tissue spaces.) Can a coal-tar derivative and known carcinogen persist in the tissue and cells of the fetus without causing harm? No one seems to have tested whether saccharin is an "active" transplacental carcinogen in the sense of causing tumors when administered only during prenatal life; but three studies have involved feeding saccharin to rats over two generations. Exposure of the second generation commenced in the womb. The higher incidence of bladder cancer in the prenatally exposed generation, Dr. Samuel Epstein comments in *The Politics of Cancer,* is a "warning of the increased sensitivity of the embryo to the carcinogenic effects of saccharin."

In a mass consumer society, there is little way to protect the young from products in wide distribution, which, like saccharin, may be purchased from the corner grocery and vending machines alike. Since fetuses are not going to learn to read warning labels, it seems that adults, however reluctantly, will have to include children and the unborn in their regulatory thinking.

It has been said that most carcinogenic exposures during fetal life probably contribute to the rate of adult cancer. Still, it is hard to avoid the suspicion that at least some cancer initiated in the womb takes its toll in childhood. The trouble is that epidemiology is so expensive—and the number of childhood cancer deaths relatively so few—that undertaking giant studies to identify possible agents of childhood cancer does not really seem to be justified. There are, however, a few situations among human children that do stand out as deserving of research and attention. The first concerns cigarettes. In two separate studies—one a combined Canadian and English investigation, and the other the Boston Epidemiology Unit analysis of the Collaborative Perinatal Project children—which embrace some 100,000 children, there has been a strange nuance in the cancer rates of those young people whose mothers smoked during the pregnancy: the childen of mothers who had smoked less than a pack a day of cigarettes had double to triple the cancer rate of children whose mothers smoked more than a pack a day. Although the total cancer rate among children of smoking mothers was somewhat higher than that of nonsmoking mothers, the Canadians concluded that smoking during pregnancy probably did not cause childhood cancer. "If maternal smoking were causally associated with childhood cancer," they commented, "one would expect to find the highest cancer rates among the offspring of the heaviest smokers."

But is this the logical expectation? Considering the large number of their pregnancies which end in miscarriage or stillbirths, heavy smokers may well lose any of their children most vulnerable to the toxic caress of cigarettes before they live long enough to officially enter the world of cancer statistics. The logic of cigarettes causing some juvenile cancers also receives support from the laboratory where benzo(a)pyrene, a component of cigarette smoke, has proven itself an enthusiastic transplacental carcinogen in animals. Smoking, of course, hardly needs more evidence on any front to condemn it as being lethal during pregnancy; but careful substantiation of human transplacental carcinogenicity might be the final straw that would make more mothers think twice.

Something about which doctors might think twice is anesthesia. Today, general surgery on pregnant women, with its accompanying exposure to inhalation anesthetics, is usually confined to medical emergencies. But pregnant women, and, by extension, their babies, still routinely encounter local anesthesia for many reasons, not the least of these being exposure during labor itself. The sole epidemiologial information anywhere about local anesthetics and childhood cancer seems, once again, to be contained in the Boston Epidemiology Analysis of the Collaborative Perinatal population. In that survey, two children out of almost three hundred prenatally exposed to the local anesthetic lidocaine during the first half of pregnancy developed malignant tumors. (Lidocaine is often used by dentists and, until a few years ago, was highly favored by obstetricians for use during labor and delivery.) Although the relative tumor risk to the lidocaine children was almost double that of other children in the study, the numbers exposed were so small that the result could easily represent a fluke or chance. Something more suspicious is that of the eight children who developed central nervous system tumors, four were prenatally exposed to procaine. (Probably most, if not all exposures to procaine, a local anesthetic more commonly known as novocain, occurred during dental work.) These are numbers which would seem to invite more investigation.

✻

Most carcinogens are not controlled by parents or by physicians. They are, instead, ubiquitous in the environment. In 1976, a group of biochemists at the University of New Orleans became curious about just what toxins and industrial compounds were reaching the contemporary fetus. Using gas chromatographic-mass spectrometry, they identifed more than 100 volatile organic chemicals in the umbilical-cord blood of a group of newborns. The list included food additives, plastics components (some of these had leached from the tubing or bag when the mother was given an intravenous), and several carcinogens. The news was even more stern when they compared these results with a gas chromato-graphic-mass spectrometry readout on the mothers' blood. Evidently some very toxic compounds, including benzene, carbon tetrachloride, and chloroform, have a preferential attraction for the fetus. The level of these substances in the newborns' blood was equal to, or higher than, the level found in maternal blood.

The New Orleans group was never able to obtain funding from the National Cancer Institute—or elsewhere—to proceed with the next step of actually breaking down the fetal chemical load to precise parts per million or billion of each chemical. Presumably, broken down in these terms, the exposure level would have been relatively low; chance, however, hardly lies with the hope that none of the known carcinogens found in the blood of these infants met its required enzyme. Chance, instead, lies with the probability that some transplacental damage took place.

With the passage of time and the continuing study of the delayed effects of ionizing radiation in man, two trends have become evident regarding tumorigenesis: more tissues have been found to be susceptible to the development of radiation-induced neoplasia and lower levels of radiation have been found to be associated with these effects.

DR. CHARLOTTE SILVERMAN
in *Preventive Medicine*

Chapter 6

# MORE THAN ENOUGH RADIATION

In the late 1950s, the world was much preoccupied with the drifting mushroom clouds left by the aboveground testing of atomic weapons. Like many people, Mary Meyer found herself wondering what exposure to fallout meant for the health of her own children and the planet. "I kept thinking," she remembers, "how could you show whether this was affecting people? One day, I was discussing it with a friend who is a radiation biologist. He said that because the female egg is so sensitive to radiation during some stages of gestation, that you should really look at the later reproductive life of girls who had been prenatally exposed to fallout or radiation. He thought this would be a very sensitive indicator of damage. Well, I just laughed," says Mary Meyer with a curt smile. "A study like that involves three generations of people. How could you ever get to do it?"

Years later, as an associate professor of epidemiology at Johns Hopkins, Mary Meyer did do this study—but not on women prenatally exposed to fallout. She did it on women who had been exposed to radiation when their mothers were X-rayed during the pregnancy. The results of this work, which is still ongoing, are among the most striking epidemiological reports in the medical literature. The evidence moves beyond a single myopic concern, such as cancer or mutation, to present a unique record of the general consequences to life and health of X-raying the fetus.

Prenatal X rays remain a stubborn component of Western obstetrics, despite much editorializing against the practice. Until the late 1950s, some doctors and hospitals routinely X-rayed all pregnant women, usually when labor started, "just in case" something was wrong. Presumably this X-raying had ended in the 1950s with the realization that X rays might cause cancer; the British, however, to their total dismay, recently found that, in eight large hospitals surveyed, abdominal X rays of one type or another were still being taken, on average, in 23 percent of deliveries, a figure pronounced "not acceptable" and in huge excess of the very few pregnancies that give clinical signs of being in trouble. The last major American survey of X rays during pregnancy, taken in 1963, found that 10 percent of pregnant women had received abdominal irradiation. A more recent but small survey, published in 1975 and covering sixteen hospitals in New York State, found that the rate of X-ray pelvimetry alone at these institutions varied from 2 percent to 16 percent of pregnancies. (X-ray pelvimetry, a procedure used to evaluate the relative size of the maternal pelvis and fetal head, is the most common reason for prebirth X rays and probably now accounts for at least three quarters of fetal exposures to ionizing radiation.)

Meyer first wanted to know whether the delicate fetal eggs could be injured for life, impairing the ability of yet unborn children to have healthy children of their own later; and second, whether direct health effects to the fetus extended beyond the small cancer risk usually thought of as the only important drawback to prenatal X rays. Various animal and human findings, Meyer commented, held out the twisted promise that "late manifestations of prenatal X-ray exposure [to the female] . . . might include growth retardation, mental retardation, hormonal changes manifested as menstrual problems and ovarian cysts, differences in general health and longevity as well as particular diseases, and effects on the brain and nervous system manifested by changes in behavior and personality." These "late manifestations" had been mainly seen, however, in little mice or in humans, such as the Hiroshima and Nagasaki survivors, who had been exposed to very high radiation doses. Few radiation biologists would have suspected it possible that a "low-level" exposure from diagnostic X rays might cause similar health problems.

Professor Meyer was able to do the "low-level" study because, in the 1960s, other Johns Hopkins researchers, working on the question of cancer and prenatal X rays, had amassed information on 20,000 X-rayed pregnant women and 36,000 control women who had given birth in Baltimore hospitals between 1947 and 1956. She sought out almost 1500 babies born to black women in this study—babies who were now teenagers, or in their early twenties, and beginning to have their own children. She chose black women simply because more of them were likely to be still living in Baltimore and accessible, and because they start having children earlier in life than white women generally do, a birth pattern that might quickly highlight any problems—and it did. By 1969, these young black women had had 15 percent more pregnancies than a carefully matched control group of non-X-rayed Baltimore black women. In the next five years, the X-rayed women, by then ranging in age from twenty-two to twenty-eight, had 7 percent more pregnancies than the control women.

At high doses, radiation is well known to kill oocytes, leaving females less fertile, or even sterile. On the other hand, radiation—which, of course, is both a cause of cancer and a cancer treatment—can have quite contradictory effects by dose. In animal experiments, relatively low radiation doses, instead of immediately destroying oocytes, have been observed to stimulate the "late stage oocytes"—those closest to maturing—to ovulate sooner than normal. This mechanism, known as "superovulation," temporarily causes radiated mother animals to give birth to more young per litter and could explain the higher fertility of the X-rayed Baltimore women.

Superovulation, however, does not appear to be without a price. In animals, a high rate of malformed offspring accompanies it. The prenatally radiated Baltimore women, with their added pregnancies, gave birth to more live children than did the nonexposed women—but they also experienced somewhat more miscarriages and had, by 1978, accumulated almost triple the fetal deaths of the control mothers. In animals, moreover, superovulation is followed by diminished fertility and then by premature sterility, the seeming consequences of the radiation's killing the female's least mature oocytes even while "stimulating" more mature ones. The excess fertility of these Baltimore women had markedly decreased over time; but whether they were destined for outright sterility in the natural course of events may never be known. By the time they were twenty-eight, almost 10 percent of the prenatally X-rayed women had had themselves surgically sterilized. Apparently, they were fed up at so often finding themselves pregnant against their own efforts at birth control.

The general health of the X-rayed women was also problematic. As they approached their thirties, it was poorer than that of the controls—although not always in statistically significant ways. More X-rayed women had, for example, left school before graduating. Not surprisingly, the major reason for their having dropped out was that they were pregnant; but more of their number had also left for reasons of "physical and social disability" and a few more of them had died over the years. A statistically significant and very telling difference was that 8 percent more X-rayed women had experienced menstrual problems severe enough that they sought medical attention for them. Their menstrual problems may well be related to the fetal deaths seen among their children. Although radiation is an undoubted mutagen, it would have to be many times more powerful than any animal or human studies have even hinted to have caused, in the diagnostic-dose range, enough lethal mutations to account for the fetal deaths among the children in Meyer's population. A similar reproductive fiasco, however, in which the female children of irradiated mother mice could not, in turn, give live birth to the children they had conceived, has been seen in the laboratory. With the mice, too, the fetal deaths were beyond those mutation could account for. The suggestion has been made that these difficult mouse pregnancies occurred because the radiation had upset the maternal "hormonal milieu."

The Meyer study slashed through a lot of accepted thinking about X rays. In the lexicon of radiology, doses below ten rads (*rad* stands for "*r*adiation *a*bsorbed *d*ose" and measures the X-ray energy absorbed per gram of tissue) are sometimes referred to as "low level." Diagnostic procedures rarely involve doses over five rads, usually do not reach beyond one or two rads, and are widely thought to be a trivial health hazard. That Meyer had observed evident systemic effects from diagnostic doses was something new and startling; yet, by comparison to the shocked response to the first studies of prenatal X rays and childhood cancer, the reaction to her work was muted. It was as though a distant cousin had come to visit. If the toxic effect is not cancer—even if the effects include fetal deaths, menstrual difficulties, swings in fertility, and an evident predisposition to general ill health—it is simply hard to interest people.

Radiation first became an extra presence in human affairs in 1895 when the German physicist Wilhelm Conrad Roentgen discovered X rays. It was almost immediately apparent that this new tool of science and medicine, while in the miracle class—or perhaps *because* it was in the miracle class—would be problematic. Before the century was over, Clarence Dally, a young assistant working with Thomas Edison on the development of X-ray equipment, died of cancer, the lesions on his radiation-burned skin having changed from ulcerous to malignant. It was also evident that medicine could hardly bring itself to concede that anything that holds the benefits X rays do when used properly could also be used wrongly.

There seems to be almost a subconscious pact about radiation studies. In the ordinary course of events, people in the Western world receive the vast majority of their exposure to ionizing radiation in the form of diagnostic X rays. In the United States, X rays account for more than 90 percent of the general population's dose of human-generated radiation—at least 20,000 times the radiation let loose on all Americans by the production of nuclear power. The remainder of human-initiated exposures are scattered among such sources as uranium mining, medical therapy, fallout from weapons-testing, and leakage from color TV sets, pacemakers, and other devices. A certain amount of natural background radiation also emanates from both the earth and from space. The average annual exposure to natural radiation in the United States is about the equivalent of, say, a spinal X ray.

In the ordinary course of radiation research, however, diagnostic X rays are about the last thing studied. This is not to say radiation is not studied at all. On the contrary, it is probably the single most researched environmental agent. More mice, more hamsters, more monkeys, and more fruit flies have been sacrificed to it than many other known hazards combined, and books and articles about these experimental probings jam the journals and overflow from the library shelves. But the follow-up of human beings exposed to diagnostic X rays has been so slight that the Meyer study represents the sole long-term study of the general consequences of the prenatal X rays to which so many babies are still routinely exposed.

In the absence of deliberate follow-up, adverse news about

radiation has often come in the ugly form of after-effects so severe that they could not be overlooked. Physicians who, in their initial pleasure with X-ray equipment, took many pictures of themselves and hardly gave a thought to radiation protection, were well represented among the first X-ray casualties. The first group of people to really force a reevaluation of X-ray usage, however, were children subjected to various sorts of high-dosage therapy. Most of these children are adults who are still alive today and, like the DES children, they are in various stages of being "recalled," like some misbegotten automobile, to have their parts looked over.

From about 1930 through the early 1960s, vogues for treating juvenile ills with high-dose X-ray "therapy" seemed to pass through medical practice as quickly as Betty Boop dolls, Mickey Mouse watches, and Hula Hoops passed through American childhood. Ringworm of the scalp became an early radiation target. The technique was just to completely burn off—or, in radiation slang, to "zap"—the child's hair. Warts and teenage acne were other radiation targets. The zenith of childhood "therapy" however, came in the 1940s and 1950s when medicine seems to have been almost hypnotized by the idea that anything that flared up around the head or neck region of the young—whether tonsils, adenoids, or the thymus gland—should be radiated into submission. Probably one million or more children were subjected to these procedures. Before World War II and the antibiotic era, radiating the tonsils or adenoids did have the justification that inflammation of these places held a risk of dangerous ear infections and operating held its own risk of infection. And, while there were other ways to treat ringworm, it did attain epidemic levels in some parts of the United States and other countries. On the other hand, radiating the thymus seems to have been "just one of those illusory ideas," in the comment of Dr. Leslie De Groot of the University of Chicago Thyroid Study Unit, "which turned out to serve no purpose."

The problem was that some of the radiation also hit the thyroid, a gland attached to the front of the larynx and now recognized as one of the most radiation-sensitive spots in the body. Apparently about 5 to 7 percent of these children are destined to get thyroid cancer, with the latency period running about five to ten years after thymus irradiation and twenty-five years or more after tonsil or adenoid therapy. The sheer number of cases has made short work of the usual quibbling about whether there is an association; in the early 1970s, for example, the University of Chicago was astonished to find that fully 1 percent of its own medical students were being treated for thyroid tumors; they represented the grown-up products of the tonsil irradiation that had been very popular in that city.

Nor is cancer the sole problem in the path of some of these radiation-exposed children. Those who received a high dose to their thymus, a gland involved in the development of the immune system, have a later disease pattern that includes a 40 percent higher rate of asthma than their own brothers and sisters and about triple the incidence of rare immunological disorders along the lines of myasthenia gravis and lupus erythematosus. (In the latter, in a sort of self-cannibalism, the body mistakes its own cells for invaders to be destroyed.) The very high head doses to the ringworm children—300 to 700 rads or more—seems to have shown itself in an increase of mental disorders. By their early twenties, these children have a somewhat higher incidence of schizophrenia, anxiety, tension headaches, and other mental problems than children whose ringworm was treated in some other fashion. Since the types of disorders are so disparate, it is thought that "radiation does not trigger a specific form of psychopathology [but may] inch subjects closer to the threshold of that type of mental illness toward which they were already predisposed."

As have the DES children, the head-and-neck-radiation children have presented something of a quandary about appropriate treatment and follow-up. Since thyroid cancer is usually easy to deal with surgically and is rarely fatal, most physicians seem to prefer just to monitor these patients for lumps or thyroid enlargement. Others have opted for the use of "thyroid replacement hormone," which, by relieving the thyroid of its own hormone-making responsibilities, shrivels it to a size unlikely to provide a haven for cancer cells. As has also been the case for the DES children, however, reassurance about the generally low risk of dying has not fully set to rest individual fears and turmoil. Dr. De Groot sometimes wonders whether "recalling these people hasn't created more anxiety than anything else."

For Susan Braudy, an attractive, lively writer who lives in New York City, the aftermath of the tonsil irradiation she had when she was eight has been a merry-go-round of conflicting medical advice and treatment proposals—a merry-go-round probably bound to keep turning until there is enough follow-up of this population to more fully quantify their risks. Ms. Braudy first realized she might have a problem when, in 1974, she came across a *New York Times* article telling about the cancer prospects for children who had once had tonsil irradiation. She remembers very clearly the strange contrast between the "neutral language of this news article" and her own swirling thoughts of immediate death. Ms. Braudy also had more than usual cause for complaint. Her tonsils were irradiated well into the antibiotic era and after she, herself, had already had a tonsillectomy, she was told the roots were growing back in.

Her first referral to the Nuclear Medicine Department of New York Hospital was a disconcerting event. She recalls that she and a friend who accompanied her were the only two people in the waiting room who were standing on their own feet. The other patients were all very pale-looking people, in wheelchairs or on stretchers, seemingly involved in last-ditch radiation treatment for cancer. She was also bothered by the thought that the radiation experts there, although now part of what New York Hospital called a "Nuclear Medicine Department" instead of an "X-Ray Department," probably included a lot of physicians who, twenty years previously, had been enthusiastically radiating the tonsils, adenoids, and thymuses of eight-year-olds like herself. When the Nuclear Medicine Department wanted to give her a thyroid scan, a procedure that would expose her to more radiation, she fled to a private physician. He, too, however, recommended a scan, and he further recommended thyroid replacement hormone—to both of which she finally conceded.

After a few years on replacement hormone, she had become accustomed to her situation and stopped thinking much about it when, while in Los Angeles for the summer, she ran out of thyroid pills. (The thyroid will resume functioning in their absence.) The Los Angeles doctor she asked to refill her prescription called her in some alarm. It was his opinion that the prescription dosage was way off and the extra thyroid hormone was putting as much pressure on her body as the routine consumption of amphetamines. He could "not in good conscience" give her a prescription.

When she returned to New York, she reported this conversation to both her internist and her thyroid specialist; they both told her that was "nonsense." At this point, Susan Braudy doesn't really know what she should do except take the philosophical point of view that "there's a sense in which we're all terminally ill" and not spend any more time worrying about her own thyroid.

For the medical profession, meanwhile, perhaps the true surprise to come from these children has not been the fact of cancer—but the extremely low doses to the thyroid associated with an excess of tumors. In 1974, the Tel Aviv University School of Medicine reported that Israeli children irradiated for ringworm between 1949 and 1969 had, over the years, developed sixfold more thyroid malignancies than their own brothers and sisters. In the Israeli estimate, a mean of only 6.5 rads had penetrated to the thyroids of these children during their scalp treatments. In 1974, it was still considered so unlikely that doses this low could cause such a large excess of cancer that the Israelis suggested their estimate might be in error; since then, doctors at New York University have estimated the mean thyroid dose to a group of New York City children irradiated for ringworm was 6 rads. Although there have been no actual cancer cases among these children, many had had surgery to remove thyroid growths of a type that could have turned malignant in time.

High-dose radiation therapy is now considered too dangerous

to use except in the treatment of diseases, such as cancer, that are themselves life-threatening. These thyroid estimates, however, assigned a very large tumor excess to doses in the low-level, or diagnostic, range. Considering the promiscuous use of diagnostic X rays in the United States, any cancer risk in this range is no small matter. In 1970, the United States Public Health Service had reported that Americans undertook 180 million patient visits a year that involved medical or dental X rays. While these figures have not been specifically updated, the Bureau of Radiological Health has estimated that by 1977 the combined total rose to 242 million patient visits. Nuclear medicine, which employs internally administered radiopharmaceuticals to diagnose and treat disease, is evidently increasing at an even faster clip. In a recent pilot study at six hospitals, the Bureau of Radiological Health learned that the use of nuclear medicine procedures was increasing by an average of 17 percent a year. The internal doses associated with nuclear medicine may be rather hefty. The estimated dose to the thyroid from various scans and "uptake" procedures, for example, ranges from about $1/10$ rad to more than 100 rads.

The idea of cancer induction at very low levels was not, however, entirely without warning. As it happens, studies of prenatal radiation and childhood cancer had long before suggested that the cancer consequences from diagnostic X rays were greater than generally assumed.

In 1956, as part of an exhaustive search for the causes of childhood cancer, Dr. Alice Stewart, who is now retired as the chairman of the Department of Social Medicine at Oxford University, undertook the first epidemiological study of a population exposed to diagnostic X rays. In the course of her researches, Dr. Stewart learned that, of children who died of leukemia before age ten, almost twice as many had been prenatally exposed to radiation (their mothers were X-rayed during the pregnancy) as had normal children.

As an individual risk, these did not translate into large numbers. Based on more complete data that followed, it has been estimated that after a prenatal exposure to 2 rads—a dosage often, although not always, sustained during pelvic or abdominal examinations—one child in every two thousand will develop leukemia; this compares with a "natural" leukemia rate of one in three thousand among white American children. What gave Stewart's report its impact was that the routine use of prenatal radiation, in both England and the United States, had spread this slight risk to literally millions of children. Stewart's preliminary 1956 dispatch to the *Lancet* fell on medicine like a black fate. Stewart, herself, estimated that, at the time, prenatal radiation had become the latent factor behind 6 or 7 percent of childhood leukemia deaths in England. (Doses in the 1950s were quite a bit higher than is common now.)

The thought of children being struck down in the womb was, of course, an awful one. Dr. Stewart initiated a frenzy of research into prenatal X rays—studies that, by now, embrace some millions of children both in England and the United States. With rare exception, they have shown a somewhat higher cancer risk among children prenatally exposed to radiation; but, perhaps more than the bulk of the data, the convincing thing to many people has been that there is a dose-effect relationship. Stewart was able to show, for instance, that the cancer risk rose roughly in accordance with the number of X-ray pictures taken during an exam; and, over the years, as improvements in equipment and technique had lowered the dose to patients, the risk to child per individual X ray has tended to diminish. "Such a relationship," writes the eminent British radiologist Robert H. Mole, "must be considered strong evidence for the causal role of diagnostic radiography."

In the immediate aftermath of Stewart, American and British physicians alike did curb their use of prenatal X rays, and in doing so provided quite convincing evidence that most prenatal X rays had, in any case, been medically useless, providing no information important to the outcome of labor. In the eight British hospitals previously mentioned, before climbing back up to the present high levels, the use of prenatal X rays dropped from 40 percent of pregnant patients in 1955 to 11 percent in 1961; the rate of stillbirths and neonatal deaths decreased steadily throughout these years. Between 1950 and 1963, the Sloane Hospital for Women in New York City decreased its percentage of prebirth X-ray pelvimetries from 16 percent to 5 percent of pregnant women; there was no evidence the pelvimetry decrease contributed to infant deaths.

A more recent and comprehensive study finds little justification at all for X-ray pelvimetry. This study, published in the *American Journal of Roentgenology* in 1975, was based on 67,000 births at sixteen hospitals in New York State. "Since pelvimetry should be used only for comparative measurements of the fetal head and maternal pelvis in order to determine whether safe vaginal delivery is possible," the research group commented, "the fundamental question is whether the physician can make this decision more accurately and more quickly with the aid of pelvimetry than would be possible using the clinical judgment." Allowing for individual exceptions and very special cases, the answer seemed to be an almost unqualified "No." In the first place, there was "little or no consistent relationship between the pelvimetry and caesarean rates at the hospitals in the study." Neither was pelvimetry of any value in shortening the length of time women were in labor before a caesarean was resorted to; in other words, for better or worse, and whether formed quickly or slowly, a physician's own judgment of the situation predominated over the X-ray information. Finally, uniform and objective clinical considerations had little to do with whether a pelvimetry was ordered at all. The main factors in ordering a pelvimetry, and exposing the fetus to radiation, were "physician-related factors"—things like the customs of the particular hospital and the experience of the physician.

In England, despite the way the use of prenatal X rays has climbed back up as the original shock from Stewart has faded, it is generally accepted that some cancer does follow from these exposures. In the United States, there is some belief—and still much argument. One objection is that pregnancies selected for X rays are already different from the norm in a way that, in itself, could predispose cancer. People, however, have looked and not been able to find any link between cancer and the common complications of pregnancy given as reasons for an X ray; and, of course, the bulk of prenatal radiation seems just to be routine rather than being ordered for "uniform and objective clinical considerations." Another objection is that children prenatally exposed to the atomic bombings did not develop an excess of childhood cancer; but the bomb population is not strictly analogous. So many of the bomb children exposed in the third trimester of gestation died within a year of being born—apparently victims to just the physical shock of the bombs or the war-torn times—that their "real" cancer rate cannot be computed.

Twenty years after Stewart, medical journals still devote an amazing effort to analyzing and reanalyzing the prenatal data. Stewart's report left the medical profession to collectively act the character of a Lady Macbeth, roaming the hallways of its past errors, paralyzed by the vision of blood on its hands. This is to everyone's misfortune. By now, although they may argue over the precise risk—whether it is one in 2,000 or 3,000 or 4,000—people who can accept the prenatal findings already do; studying another few million children won't convince the rest. Meanwhile, there are other things to be found out about radiation.

Some people, for example, do not believe the prenatal studies contain a general warning about diagnostic radiation because the fetus is uniquely sensitive to radiation; others are not so sure the fetus stands unique before radiation. The available studies, while perhaps not conclusive, imply a continuing measure of risk that is larger for children than grown-ups. A major American study, for example, came to the interesting conclusion that when children were X-rayed at two sites in their bodies, in doses that are considered truly trivial (as in the teeth and extremities), they did incur a slightly greater leukemia risk; there seemed to be a combined impact.

In 1978, Dr. Rosalie Bertell, then at the Roswell Park Memorial Institute in Buffalo, thought to look at the question a bit differently. She found that every past exposure to one rad of trunk or abdominal radiation decreased by a year the age at which men tended to develop nonlymphatic leukemias. While the nonlymphatic leukemias are known to be particularly radiation-sensitive, and this a-year-per-rad equation may not apply to other cancer types, the Bertell study is yet again a reminder that the body stores away radiation exposures like bad memories; the younger in life these exposures occur, the larger, of course, the chance the latent memory will surface to haunt an individual.

Cancer is hardly the single worrisome aspect of radiation exposures—especially exposures to the fetus. The Meyer study stands out like a huge, lonely arrow, pointing toward other damage worth confirming and other dangers worth understanding; after all, that eight more women in any one hundred prenatally exposed to X rays may later find themselves with nagging menstrual problems seems as good a reason to avoid "routine" X-ray pelvimetries as the chance that one in three or four thousand of them will develop cancer. Dr. Robert Miller, meanwhile, has concerned himself about another system that may be very radiation-sensitive—the delicate fetal nervous system.

Dr. Miller, interestingly, is prominent among American scientists not convinced of the carcinogenicity of prenatal X rays. "I just don't see it," he says. On the other hand, he also dissents from the idea that cancer is the only "real" index of environmental harm. He has been studying the head size of children prenatally exposed to the atomic bombs, and has found that the head size of rather large numbers of them is smaller than normal—a sign the radiation has stunted their brain growth. While it was not unexpected that prenatal exposure to the bombs would stunt growth in many ways, the small doses associated with small head size were surprising to everyone; 10 to 19 rads of radiation carried a significant risk that the child's head and brain had been stunted. This dosage, Dr. Miller pointed out in the *Lancet*, "is the lowest yet known to produce a detectable [birth] defect in man. When [brain cell] depletion is great enough, mental retardation ensues. With less depletion, intelligence is within normal range, but may be reduced as compared with the child's full potential had he not been irradiated. It seems, therefore, that even small [prenatal] exposures may deprive the individual of some intelligence."

✳

As disturbing as the early reports of prenatal radiation and cancer may have been to physicians, for more than a decade after their appearance the debate over low-level effects was largely the obscure material of scientific journals. The first scientists to really force this debate into the open were not concerned about X rays; their concern was emission standards for nuclear power plants. In the early 1960s the Federal Radiation Council set the maximum permissible individual dose of radiation at five rads per person every "generation," or thirty years, "exclusive of natural background and the deliberate exposure of patients by practitioners of the healing arts." In other words, the Federal Radiation Council was signaling the nuclear power industry that it could count on being allowed to expose every American to this much radiation in the course of thirty years. (In 1970, the Environmental Protection Agency took over the standard-setting functions of the FRC. Although the same "permissible limit" technically remains in effect, the EPA recently lowered the maximum permissible individual exposure to radiation specifically from nuclear energy production to the equivalent of 25 millirads—a millirad is a thousandth of a rad—a year.)

Later in the decade, Dr. John W. Gofman and Dr. Arthur R. Tamplin, respectively a specialist in nuclear-physical chemistry and a biophysicist, and then both research associates at the Lawrence Radiation Laboratory in Livermore, California, came up with a much-publicized reckoning of the cancer cost of this guideline. They thought that exposing the full population to the "permissible limit" would result in 32,000 extra cancer deaths a year, or about a 10 percent increase. A national furor followed and the government was moved to recognize low-level radiation officially. The FRC commissioned the National Academy of Sciences to undertake a comprehensive investigation of radiation protection and hazards. In 1972, the Academy's Advisory Committee on the Biological Effects of Ionizing Radiation heaved forth 217 over-sized pages, officially known as "The Effects on Populations of Exposure to Low Levels of Ionizing Radiation," but usually just called the BEIR Report.

To the general wonder, the BEIR Report, in the comment of *Science*, "provided what could be alternatively read as cold comfort for the critics of Gofman and Tamplin or as a measure of vindication for the two scientists." The National Academy, which rarely sounds alarms about what science may be doing to the public, hardly quarreled with the idea of a low-level radiation threat; but it did quarrel with some of Gofman and Tamplin's underlying assumptions, saying that they had overestimated the lifetime risk from prenatal radiation and the "extra" cancer susceptibility of children. The BEIR Panel thought that between 3,000 and 15,000 extra cancer deaths would follow from exposing the full populace to the "permissible limit" for nuclear power.

But the debate over cancer deaths from nuclear power was hardly more than a footnote. In 1972, as now, the nuclear energy risks were mainly theoretical. According to the Nuclear Regulatory Commission, the average dose to each American from the production of nuclear energy in 1977 was the equivalent of one millirad. This was about $1/170$ the average annual dose that, over thirty years, would add up to the permissible limit. These figures require the qualification that the government only willingly tells about "legal" and monitored emissions from power plants. In those places where there has been leakage from plants, or from improperly stored wastes, local exposures may be higher. Still, leaving aside people employed in the nuclear power industry, it would be surprising if anyone could show that the current production of nuclear energy is exposing more than one out of a hundred Americans to as much radiation as is attendant to X-raying a single molar.

In 1972, as now, however, the millions of annual patient visits for diagnostic X rays were not theoretical. Even the scientists, physicians, and government regulators who prepared the BEIR Report, most of whom had spent their lives administering or dealing with radiation, appeared somewhat stunned when they communally considered the implications of the relentless American exposure to diagnostic X rays. Using their projections, the continuing use of diagnostic X rays at 1970 levels—of course, the use of X rays has increased by about 60 million annual patient visits since then—would, aside from the risk of mutation and other damage, eventually claim some 2600 extra cancer victims a year. (Using Gofman and Tamplin's base estimates of cancer susceptibility, the toll might be around 14,000 lives.) Eighty years after X rays were discovered to be carcinogenic and forty-five years after they were discovered to be mutagenic, the government had issued its first substantial warning that their diagnostic use involved some hazard. Moreover, no matter whose base estimates were used, the point was that these estimates of the danger of diagnostic X rays were still largely being interpolated from other data rather than from studying the later health history of X-rayed patients. In 1972, virtually the only direct studies of low-level radiation were still the studies of prenatal X rays and childhood cancer launched in the wake of Stewart's studies.

The lateness of the warning and the essential flimsiness of the data served to point out the government's compromised position on radiation. X rays, after all, are the only medical device whose basic components are also used to formulate atomic bombs and as a very controversial energy source. Bad news about radiation strikes too many raw nerves at once—the Defense Department, the medical and dental professions, the nuclear power industry— for the government to welcome it on any level. Not only has the government failed to sponsor appropriate back-up studies for a device as widely used as X-ray machines, equally important, there has been no area of scientific research that has seen scientists more quickly punished for finding—and loudly announcing—adverse data. In a 1978 testimony to the House Subcommittee on Health and the Environment, Dr. Tamplin described how the Atomic Energy Commission had blocked his work and made him a "nonperson" after his complaints about nuclear energy. In similar fashion, Dr. Irwin Bross, the chief biostatistician at Roswell Park Memorial Institute, the nation's oldest cancer research center, a few years ago complained that the National Cancer Institute was exposing women under age fifty to a foolhardy cancer risk by enrolling large numbers of them in experimental breast-cancer screening programs that included an annual mammogram, or breast X ray; the National Cancer Institute revoked the funding it had supplied Roswell Park for nine years—and with this move ended one of the very few research programs anywhere that focused on damage from diagnostic X rays. Actually, not even a Nobel Prize has proven to be protection against such harassment. In 1955, for example, the United States delegation to the Geneva "Atoms for Peace" Conference exquisitely embarrassed itself by, at the last moment, forbidding Dr. Herman Muller, the geneticist who had discovered the mutagenicity of X rays, to deliver his scheduled talk on the adverse effects of radiation.

In the absence of direct data about X-rayed populations, virtually all "accepted" medical ideas about the hazards of diagnostic radiation have come from interpreting animal data or from the follow-up of Hiroshima and Nagasaki survivors. For many reasons, the Hiroshima and Nagasaki survivors are a troubling population on which to base conclusions about diagnostic X rays. The great problem of interpretation they present is simply that all radiation is not alike; radiation impact differs by various "quality factors"— as radiation science puts it—including the type of radiation used and the time sequence of doses. The Hiroshima bomb, for example, contained a large component of fast neutrons. One result of this was that even though the radiation "dose" to Hiroshima was smaller than that to Nagasaki, Hiroshima victims have manifested both a higher cancer rate and a different ratio of cancer types than seen in Nagasaki. To compare the effects of this neutron-dominated radiation with X rays requires a calculation of the Relative Biological Effectiveness (RBE) of the two radiation types. The appropriate RBE for various radiation effects at various radiation dosages is a subject still mired in disagreement among radiation scientists. Also, a given amount of radiation spread out over time does not entail the same genetic, cancer, and other risks as the same amount received in a single blast from a bomb. This differential, too, has to be estimated, argued, and factored into the equation.

Doses modified by "quality factors" are expressed in rems (*r*oentgen *e*quivalent *m*an) rather than rads. This convention signals that the dose under discussion does not come directly from X-ray studies but has been recalculated or modified in some way to render it the presumed equal of a rad. A way of looking at this idea is that a certain number of British pounds (rads) and another, different number of American dollars (rems) will buy the same amounts of cognac (biological damage) on the open market any one day. The difference is that some international banking computer has determined the precise currency exchange acceptable that day; health physicists, on the other hand, are not in complete agreement about the "quality factors" appropriate for converting the neutron-dominated Hiroshima radiation into rems—or the presumed equivalent of an X-ray rad.

To Dr. Bross, to start with these conversions is to start backwards. "The health physicists," he objects, "go through a completely different process than we do. They try to guess about the dose to the bomb victims and guess again about the Relative Biological Effectiveness of various radiation sources. Well, if you guess wrong at any stage, the whole thing is off. In epidemiology you have solid, base data. You take a population. You know they had this many X rays. This or that happened to them. I have to say I'm really sick of the other way."

Between the Hiroshima data and the relatively sparse diagnostic data, people are arguing about whether their colleagues' estimates of cancer risks are perhaps fifty times too low or too high; these differences actually look tidy by comparison with the mutation disputes. There, people are arguing whether their colleagues' estimates of the radiation damage to the DNA ensconced in sperm and eggs may be 100 to 500 times off the mark. This is not to say that the Hiroshima data is necessarily all "incorrect" and the diagnostic data is all "correct." Human epidemiology on any subject is, of course, full of pitfalls. It is to say, however, that there has hardly been a proper and unhampered scientific effort to reconcile the divergent data on so crucial a topic. No one, after all, expected much good from atomic bombs in the first place. Diagnostic X rays, by contrast, are a great advance and benefit when properly used. The misfortune is that trustworthy guidelines for their proper and appropriate use are still not to be had.

Radiation is among the strongest mutagens to which people are routinely exposed. Perhaps the most depressing information to come from the 1970 Public Health Survey was that shielding of patients' reproductive organs had been used, as the Bureau of Radiological Health later commented, "in only a small percentage of the examinations" for which this procedure "could be considered appropriate." Described by one radiologist as "the most important thing you can do for a patient you are X-raying," shielding with lead aprons, blocks, or other devices minimizes the dose to the reproductive organs. The Bureau of Radiological Health considers shielding "appropriate" when the primary beam directly strikes the gonads or comes within five centimeters of them. Simply because of the out-of-the-way location of the penis and scrotum, shielding is easier to carry out on men; for them it usually negates about 90 percent of mutational risk of radiation. Shielding the ovaries is sometimes possible, but often would obstruct the X-ray picture.

In any case, to judge from the 1970 figures, whether easy or not, talk about shielding was largely academic in the minds of most radiologists and their technicians (or, as they are now called, "technologists"). They simply weren't doing it. The situation may have changed in response to the great emphasis on shielding that has since characterized the Bureau of Radiological Health's educational programs. Or the situation may not have changed. In 1974, in a burst of enthusiasm for shielding, the American College of Radiologists distributed a lead-lined athletic cup—or "shaped contact shield," as they delicately termed it—to every radiologist in the country. Contact shields could hardly be easier to use; but it is the impression of a Bureau of Radiological Health official that "75 percent of them are gathering dust in closets." The problem is that few radiologists now take X-ray pictures themselves; their work is confined to "reading" the results. The job of taking pictures has been assigned to technologists, the majority of whom are young and female. "Well, they get embarrassed," explains the Radiological Health official. "They just don't want to hand a shield to some guy."

Meanwhile, the argument rages about the mutational danger attached to X rays. Americans sustain the highest annual "genetically significant dose"—the average X-ray dose to a citizenry's reproductive organs—of any people in the world. Is the year-in, year-out contact with diagnostic radiation noticeably compromising future children and even now perhaps silently condemning them to early deaths, or malformations, or just nagging diseases? "Experimental studies," Dr. Miller commented in 1974, "provide overwhelming evidence that radiation is mutagenic. Man is probably no exception." This may be the only noncontroversial statement that could be made about radiation and mutation.

Technically, mutation is defined as "any change in the genetic material." For practical purposes, two broad categories of mutation present themselves: chromosomal disorders and point mutations. The first category embraces abnormalities in the chromosomes, the long filamentous structures in the cell nucleus to which the genes are affixed. Each human cell has forty-six chromosomes (with the exception of the germ cells, which possess twenty-three chromosomes), half supplied by the mother's egg and half from the father's sperm. The fact that perhaps half of spontaneously aborted fetuses are chromosomally abnormal suggests, of course, that breaks, reshuffling, deletions, and other chromosome damage occurs fairly often in the germ cells and that such damage is more often than not fatal to a fetus formed from these cells.

Each chromosome, in turn, contains thousands and thousands of genes, the specific portions of DNA that control each recognizable trait of the living organism. In the genes reside decisions about the more superficial boundaries of life—such as hair color, height, and body shape—and about the fundamental terms on which a life will be lived. Changes in the structure of the genes are known as point mutations, and their influence on health may range from being lethal early in fetal existence, to arousing major disease along the lines of diabetes, schizophrenia, and sickle cell anemia, to the "imperceptible loss of vigor and vitality" Crow warned about. While chromosomal aberrations may loom larger under the microscope, it is point mutations that loom largest for mankind. In any acceleration of the mutation rate, "small" point mutations, the ones that nag at health and well-being, are thought to easily outweigh "drastic ones which produce fatal hereditary diseases and spectacular malformations." It is in their ostensible "mildness" that their ultimate danger lies. The Environmental Mutagen Society has emphasized that "point mutations are likely to allow the afflicted individuals to survive and reproduce, and may thus be transmitted and affect subsequent generations. In terms of human suffering, therefore, the summed effects of single gene mutations probably exceed the deleterious effects of changes in chromosome number or arrangement."

Point mutations, in short, are the great mystery and key to life and the great focus of genetic research; they are also, however, the mutational event hardest to monitor with the clumsy tools presently available. Only damage to the chromosomes is large enough to be picked up under the microscope. Wonderfully precise analysis of the chemical composition of the genes promises to be the technique that will soon allow for point mutations in whole populations to be monitored. At present, however, ideas about the amount of mutation, and "human suffering," attributable to radiation have been drawn mainly from animal work and from monitoring human diseases that might represent point mutations.

The technique for measuring lethal and very damaging point mutations in animals and insects is to radiate them and then measure survival rates, abnormalities, fertility, and other fairly obvious indices of health among their offspring. But animals and insects are of virtually no help in measuring point mutations that may contribute to anxiety, depression, tiredness, allergy, and other small conditions humans would rather be without. As the BEIR Panel emphasized, far from being able to detect small or subtle mutations in experimental studies, it is not even known what aspects of animal or insect health would "perhaps be the human counterparts of these mutations . . . causing a slight reduction in life expectancy . . . greater susceptibility to disease, impaired physical or mental vigor, or a slight malformation of some organ. . . . We cannot," the Panel dryly noted, "ask a drosophila [fly] if it has a headache."

Theoretically, of course, one could ask the offspring of humans exposed to radiation if they have headaches. But, in practice, trying to measure vague or lesser human ills is a task of almost self-defeating subtlety. (What, after all, is the "normal" incidence of headache?) As a practical matter, human monitoring for the genetic effects of radiation is also pretty much confined to watching the offspring of radiated parents for health problems that are easily identified—problems along the lines of stillbirth, early death, and major malformations. Almost nothing is known about the radiation-induction of those point mutations that are probably the most important in terms "of human suffering . . . allow[ing] the afflicted individuals to survive and reproduce." And even major signs, such as infant death and malformation, have not cooperated in showing a uniform induction in all populations studied.

The largest human group ever monitored for signs of radiation-caused genetic damage is the children of atomic bomb survivors. The "genetic group"—as distinct from the limited group of children *in utero* at the time of the bombings—includes all children both conceived and born after the bombings. It now runs to thousands of people. (Actually, the first generation of this group will not be complete until all Japanese exposed to the bombs, however young they were at the time, are themselves past reproductive age.)

There was intense worry that the postbomb children would include large numbers of genetic freaks who were sickly, malformed, and died young. Until 1952, the Atomic Bomb Casualty Commission, a joint Japanese-American body that has studied the health aftermath of the bombings,* monitored nearly all children born to bomb survivors for six "genetic indices"—including such things as the youngsters' malformations, neonatal deaths, and stillbirths—that might confirm severe damage to their parents' genes. To the surprise of most people involved, there did not seem to be anything notably wrong with these children. By 1952, when 77,000 postbomb children had been born and there was no significant difference between their health and the health of children whose parents were not in Hiroshima or Nagasaki at the time of the bombings, the ABCC decided monitoring for the six "genetic indices" was no longer necessary; it confined its genetic-damage monitoring to a watch on the death rates of the postbomb children as they matured.

Years went by, and still nothing appeared to be wrong. The death rate of the postbomb children was not unusual. Even the more conservative radiation commentators were somewhat baffled by the apparent good health of these children. James V. Neel, the chairman of the Department of Medical Genetics at the University of Michigan and who headed much of the ABCC genetic monitoring, and his colleagues, expressed the general bewilderment. "Unless one is willing to argue that man differs from all other forms of life thus far studied," they commented in 1966, "lethal and semilethal mutations of a type which might manifest themselves in the first decade of life were induced [by the bombs]. But the present study provides no evidence for their existence."

Only in 1972—the most recent summary of results from the genetic watch—with 19,000 postbomb children having been followed, on average until they were seventeen years old, did the death rate of the postbomb children show a suspicious increase. And, even then, the difference in their rate of death only attained "borderline significance" when the father had been the exposed parent. Based on the 1972 observations, and after making the usual "quality corrections," the Neel group estimated that the

* In keeping with the public relations of the age, the ABCC recently changed its name to the more neutral Radiation Effects Research Foundation.

"doubling dose" for mutations that would kill children within the first seventeen years of life was "unlikely" to be less than 138 for men and could be as much as 1000 rems for women from radiation encountered in the form of low-level X rays. (The doubling dose is that radiation dose that doubles the chance of a natural event's occurring. While it is a convenient way for scientists to express conclusions and comparisons, it does not imply that it is all right for people to encounter that much extra radiation. The doubling dose for breast cancer, for example, would see one out of every seven, instead of the present one out of every fourteen, American women develop breast tumors.)

As Dr. Neel himself has cautioned, these numbers only apply to what are essentially "dominant lethal" mutations—those mutations that cause an offspring to die before, in turn, reaching reproductive age. In the minds of some radiation biologists, the mechanism for inducing dominant lethals is so different from other mutations that it "cannot be properly expressed" as a doubling dose. In mice, too, the doubling dose for dominant lethals extends to "very high values of several hundreds of thousands" of rems; but experimentation has shown that this does not excuse the mouse from succumbing to other crucial mutations at fractions of that dose. The doubling dose to mice that produces semi-sterility in the next generation is around 30 rems; the doubling dose for mutations that cause skeletal abnormalities is about half that.

Directly studying X-rayed human beings again has told a different story than studying bombed human beings. Available studies of the children of X-rayed parents suggest that, to the contrary, low-level radiation has sometimes been fatal and sometimes been malforming.

The classic study here may be a comparison of the families of 2000 radiologists, and almost as many other physician-specialists, which was published in 1955. Stanley Macht, then the director of the Department of Radiology at Washington County Hospital, and Philip Lawrence, then Chief of the Familial Studies Unit of the federal Public Health Service, undertook this very detailed comparison. They found that the fetal death rate of radiologists' children was 2 percent higher than that of the children of other physician-specialists; they found "a consistent trend of higher abnormality" among the radiologists' children; and they also found that the radiologists' children had a 30 percent higher rate of neoplasms—abnormal tissue growths, whether benign or malignant—than did the children of other physician-specialists. These results stand out against the fact that the control group was, in itself, hardly innocent of toxic exposures. The control physicians included many men who also dealt with radiation equipment fairly often, and it included anesthesiologists, a group of men now thought to have their own reproductive troubles. A final point of interest that Macht and Lawrence picked up was that the radiologists had had somewhat more children, and had them earlier in life, than other physicians; they were quite struck by this trend, and, as Mary Meyer would do two decades later, they proposed that "radiation effects may possibly increase fertility in the earlier [reproductive] years and cause [a] decrease only later on."

However, the real warning about X rays—and contradiction to the bomb data—has not come from studying possible signs of point mutations; it has come from studying chromosome aberrations. In human populations, of course, children with Down's syndrome are the premier omens of chromosome damage. In 1961, Irene Uchida, the Canadian investigator who was the first to point out that Down's babies are now being born to younger mothers, compared the X-ray histories of 81 mothers of Down's children with those of 81 women who had given birth to children with cleft lips. Although not able to obtain precise doses in their X-ray backgrounds, she did confirm that 23 of the mothers of Down's children had had four or more abdominal X rays; among the cleft-lip mothers, only three women had sustained this much radiation before conceiving the child in question. In 1965 at Johns Hopkins, X-ray histories were taken for 200 Down's children; it was found that seven times the number of their mothers as of control mothers had sustained "combined radiation from one or more diagnostic, fluoroscopic and therapeutic sources."

When the 1972 BEIR Report was issued, these two studies were placed against the bomb results. The bomb results, as usual, won. As there had not been an increase in the number of Down's children being born to bomb survivors, the BEIR Panel opted for the "bad seed" theory to explain the X-ray results; it suggested that the X-rayed women may have already been in poor health and that their own genetic infirmity was the cause of their children's sorry chromosomes.

In the intervening years, however, people interested in Down's syndrome and X rays have refined their data in a fashion that always adds credence to a biological proposal—they have shown a dose-effect response. In late 1972, for example, Eva Alberman, an English physician and public health specialist, compared the X-ray experiences of 465 mothers of Down's children and 465 mothers of children with other severe defects. In this group, "the mothers of those with Down's syndrome had more total X rays, both in number and dose, before conception." (Alberman has also studied the X-ray history of women who had spontaneously aborted a chromosomally abnormal embryo or fetus; in those cases, she found that the more X rays a woman had accumulated before conceiving, the more likely it was that her fetus or embryo would display a range of fatal chromosome aberrations.) Various researchers now place the radiation doubling dose for Down's syndrome at between one and 4.6 rads; these numbers, if correct, entirely contradict the idea that a few X rays here and there are genetically harmless.

A curious twist to Alberman's data may explain why no "extra" Down's children were seen in the immediate aftermath of the bomb. Both with the live Down's children she studied and with the chromosomally abnormal fetuses which had miscarried, only maternal X rays taken ten or more years before the child's conception contributed "significantly" to chromosome damage. Alberman suggests that this twist may mean radiation "accelerates oocyte aging" rather than immediately disrupting the chromosomes. The idea that radiation would accelerate the aging of oocytes is not surprising, since radiation is widely considered to have a general aging effect on the body. It is, however, an idea that makes a huge difference in comparing the bomb and X-ray results; if X rays, rather than harming the egg right away, accelerate an aging process that, a decade later, results in a chromosomal breakdown, the Atomic Bomb Casualty Commission would not have found this out. Ten years after the bombings, of course, the ABCC was no longer monitoring abnormalities and birth defects among postbomb children; it had already decided they were in such good condition that monitoring could be confined to their death rate.

This, again, is not to say the bomb findings are valueless; they have revealed a lot of the proclivities of radiation. It *is* to say that several X-ray studies, some done by people of international reputation, seriously challenge the bomb results. In view of this challenge, to constantly cite the bomb results as the court of final appeal for deciding radiation protection and hazards is not acceptable. Things have a way of coming full circle. Eva Alberman's work brings to mind a similar, strange nuance in Stewart's data. In 1958, Dr. Stewart had not only questioned the mothers of children who had died of cancer about prenatal X rays. She also thought to question them about preconceptual X rays. While the effect was not a large one—perhaps one quarter that of directly X-raying the fetus—she did learn that the more preconceptual abdominal X rays a woman had sustained, the more likely it was that her child would later develop cancer. She also learned that the farther in the past from conception, the stronger was the X-ray link to cancer in the child. In 1958, Stewart was mystified by this time sequence. Why would X rays taken years before the conception of a child be more risky than those taken months before? Alberman's ideas about oocyte aging and mutational events may provide an answer. The time sequence in both the Alberman and Stewart studies again underlines that children stand in special jeopardy before radiation. Little girls are thought of as little girls; it is hard to realize that X-raying them may cause more harm to future children than X-raying a grown woman. The human mind knows danger as an immediate thing; radiation is something that flashes and disappears. But not, apparently, for the oocyte.

*

Even through disagreements over their dangers, X rays have been enough abused that groups ranging from the Nader-founded Health Research Group to the now-defunct Federal Radiation Council, to, most recently, the Interagency Task Force on Ionizing Radiation have mounted campaigns against the situation. In general, the theme of these campaigns is that X rays should not be a routine or random part of medical practice, but taken only when pre-existing symptoms—the aching tooth, the troubled pregnancy, the broken arm—justify an exposure. Even the American Dental Association has recommended that "radiographic examinations should not be made a part of every dental examination"—in other words, no X rays every six months. Such campaigning, however, appears to have done little good. A few years ago, the FDA estimated that perhaps 30 percent of X rays are medically unnecessary. Two Massachusetts Institute of Technology researchers have further concluded that, leaving aside those 30 percent or so of medical X rays that may represent a misjudgment, another 30 percent represent no medical judgment at all; they are, instead, taken for the sole purpose of defensive medicine—that is, just to have on hand in case the physician is sued.

Protecting themselves against lawsuits that haven't even been filed yet may seem a unique way for physicians to use a known carcinogen and known mutagen; but possibly only the saints among us, if physicians, would not do the same faced with the current public frenzy for malpractice cases. The fact is, for all the agreement about X-ray abuse, no one seems to know how to force a reduction. As long ago as 1956, the National Academy of Sciences was alarmed enough to propose that there be "a national system of radiation-exposure record keeping." The thought behind the proposal was that physicians confronted with a patient whose "lifetime record" already showed many X-ray exposures might be reluctant to add to the volume. "We are conscious of the fact this recommendation will not be simple to put into effect," the Academy noted, but added that the genetic stakes justified the attempt.

Dr. Bross, and the Health Research Group, more simply

suggest that patients question their physicians about the need for every X ray. "The doctors will yell at you, of course," Bross comments, "but I can't help that." Dr. John Caffrey, Professor Emeritus of Radiology at the College of Physicians and Surgeons at Columbia University and senior author of the standard medical textbook *Pediatric X-Ray Diagnosis,* thinks about 20 to 30 percent of childhood exposures could be eliminated "without any loss of useful clinical diagnostic information" just by having the clinician and radiologist briefly discuss the need for each exposure. "In discussing roentgen examinations one would like to see pediatricians and radiologists drop such misleading phrases as 'Let's take a picture of Mary's abdomen," or 'Let's try a barium swallow,'" Caffrey goes on. "These pejorative statements actually signify that the patient is going to be flushed with ionizing radiation, and in the case of pelvic and abdominal examinations, the gonads will be in the direct rays."

Will any of this be effective? There is an element beyond logic and reason in the overuse of X rays. Perhaps they are just too lulling a cross between a child's camera and an adult toy—the big, glossy pictures, the technologist warning "Now lie completely still"—to be taken seriously. The British, after all, would take them seriously if anyone did. Their medical journals, unlike American ones, editorialize fervently against unneeded X rays; and, since the malpractice suit has yet to become a national pastime on the British Isles, it would seem that "defensive medicine" is not the reason behind many X rays there. Nonetheless it turned out that British physicians, on average, were still X-raying 23 percent of pregnant women; they also X-rayed 10 percent of newborns. A full 10 percent of the British population was being twice "flushed with ionizing radiation" before they were a week into this world.

What especially chagrined the British was that, in recent years, everyone had presumed that sonar, or sound wave equipment, by presenting a substitute way of obtaining internal images, had really slashed X-ray use during pregnancy. While not as well tested as many people, including the American Bureau of Radiological Health, would like, and while not an adequate replacement for all X-ray procedures (sonar, for example, cannot be used for pelvimetries; the thick pelvic bone "blocks" the signal) exposing the fetus to sound waves whenever possible is a great improvement over exposing the fetus to ionizing radiation. The British eight-hospital survey, however, found that physicians were now just taking *both* sonar and X-ray pictures.

"It seems," the British concluded in exasperation, "that where a patient attends a hospital with readily accessible X-ray facilities, these facilities will be used." It would seem from this conclusion that the only sure means of reducing radiation doses to the public is to improve the equipment and the techniques employed in obtaining the X-ray pictures, which physicians insist on ordering against all warning, editorials, and protest.

In 1974, the Bureau of Radiological Health took perhaps the most crucial step toward reducing doses from individual X rays— the bureau has no means of stopping physicians from taking too many X rays to begin with—by requiring that all new stationary general purpose X-ray machines be equipped with automatic collimators. These devices, by sternly restricting the size of the X-ray beam to the size of the film, eliminate the often erroneous manual adjustments of often untrained technicians.

A pediatric breakthrough, although a sad one in its necessity, is a new system marketed by the 3M Company, which uses intensifying screens and high-speed film to detect subtle bone chips and fractures in suspected cases of child abuse. Dr. Armand E. Brodeur, the chief of radiology at Cardinal Glennon Children's Hospital in St. Louis, recently told United Press International that, by using the new system, he had been able to confirm 10 percent more cases of child abuse while employing about half the radiation of conventional systems. "I don't promote medical products," Dr. Brodeur commented, "but I promote health through diagnosis. Anything that is going to give more detail and less radiation is going to help me."

Since radiation equipment is not an instamatic camera in the simplicity of its operations, the other crucial step is to improve the training of technologists. The Bureau of Radiological Health has not met with much success in trying to accomplish this. As of 1977, only four American states required that X-ray technologists be trained and licensed for their work. Although the bureau has bitterly complained to Congress that, elsewhere, people "can walk in off the street" and be hired to deal out radiation, Congress has for years declined to require national training standards. Meanwhile, surveys both in the United States and Europe have again and again confirmed that doses administered during common procedures will vary by factors of ten, twenty, and even a hundred, depending on the technologist's skills.

Aside from improvements in technique and equipment, perhaps the only other hope of adding logic to X-ray use would be to stamp every machine in the country with these observations from *Mankind Evolving,* Theodosius Dobzhansky's virtuoso book on genes and the human prospect:

> All forms of high-energy or penetrating or ionizing radiation, from the "softest" X rays to gamma rays of radium and presumably cosmic rays, increase the frequencies of mutations in all experimental organisms studied. . . . There is no minimum or safe or threshold amount of radiation below which mutations will not be induced. Any increase, however small, of the amount of radiation to which living beings are exposed will augment the numbers of mutations that arise . . . these extra, additional mutations will continue to maim and murder human beings for many generations after our present conflicts, concerns and follies will have been forgotten.

But, you know, even people that can get
pregnant have to eat.

ODESSA KOMER<br>
Vice President,<br>
United Automobile Workers

# Chapter 7

# GENES AND JOBS

The small San Joaquin Valley town of Lathrop, California, contains
about 500 people, two factories, and one post office. A few years
ago, in gossip and over lunch, it came out that none of the men
working in the pesticide section of one of those factories—the
Occidental Chemical Company's Lathrop Division—had conceived a child since coming to work there. After consultation with
their union, and some prodding by co-workers and wives, six of
these men sought sperm counts. In July 1977, the results came

190 • AT HIGHEST RISK

back; all the counts were abnormal, with some men having no sperm at all and others a level below that generally considered necessary to conceive children. At the time the counts came back, no one knew for sure what toxic exposure might be at fault. The blame, however, was soon placed on DBCP (dibromochloropropane), the pesticide ingredient that these men primarily handled and that, even though known to damage animal sperm at exposures of only a few parts per million, had been extensively applied to vegetable crops for the previous eighteen years. "We really were shocked," remembers Rex Cook, the secretary-treasurer of the Occidental local of the Oil, Chemical and Atomic Workers' Union. "Before this, I'd never even heard of DBCP."

The shock, however, was felt far beyond Lathrop. Aside from the 2,000 industrial workers and several thousand agricultural workers who had been sustaining fairly intense exposures to DBCP, probably the entire American population, and millions of other people in Canada, Mexico, and elsewhere, had also sustained fairly routine, if not daily, exposures to DBCP during the years it was in use. Checking over their own food supply later in 1977, the Canadians detected 2 parts per million of DBCP on radishes and 1.5 ppm on carrots—no small numbers for something as toxic as DBCP. While there had never been a federal standard governing DBCP, at least one major manufacturer, Dow Chemical, had set a limit of 1 ppm in air as a safe workplace exposure for its own employees. All told, reporter William K. Stevens wrote in a front-page commentary in the *New York Times*, DBCP had become "the villain in what has developed as one of the most dramatic, clear-cut and widespread instances of environmental contamination since public attention began focusing on such matters in the 1960s.

"A flock of serious questions," he further commented, "had been raised by all this." "How seriously have agricultural workers been affected, if at all? How serious is the cancer link? Can people be affected if they eat vegetables grown in soil treated with DBCP? How can everyone involved be protected?"

DBCP has now been banned and probably many of these questions will never receive an answer. Even in exile, however, DBCP has lingered like a sour taste. If as gonadotoxic an agent as

DBCP had been used in several countries for almost two decades before its effect on humans was noticed, what other gonadotoxic agents perhaps still in mass use have escaped notice? There was a level at which DBCP evoked a sort of final technological nightmare that chemical carelessness would foreclose even the possibility of reproduction. "I think people are being exposed to other things that are just as serious right now," comments Rex Cook. "But I can't prove it yet. I suppose I'll have to wait until a bunch of workers keel over dead and then say 'I told you so.' "

Continuing observation of DBCP has also shown that the same agent can have both a temporary and, apparently, a permanent impact on sperm, depending on exposure levels. Many agricultural workers who applied DBCP-containing pesticides in the fields seem, for example, to have experienced mild sperm count depressions, which disappeared within a year of their being away from the stuff; but, by mid-1979, with DBCP having been banned almost two years, factory workers with zero counts had yet to recover any fertility. The sperm of those DBCP workers who still had some have been subjected to a very interesting chromosome analysis. In sperm, the Y chromosome, which is the male sex chromosome, readily picks up a stain that renders it fluorescent and quite viewable under the microscope. Occasional errors of spermatogenesis endow a single sperm with two Y chromosomes. In normal men, the frequency of double-Y sperm seems to be about 1.2 percent; in DBCP-exposed men, this frequency triples to become 3.8 percent.

A double-Y sperm is quite capable of viable fertilization, the result being an XYY child—individuals sometimes known as "supermales." At present, about one out of a thousand male babies is an XYY child. Some people may recall that, years ago, there was a great fuss over the theory that these men, who are often taller than average, were also violent, criminal types. The theory of double-Y criminality is now seriously disputed and Y chromosome nondisjunction may be a relatively unimportant chromosome error for the individual—although perhaps not for the species. What worries biologists more is that agents that increase this easily analyzed error may also increase errors not as readily visible, or "fluorescent," under the microscope. Dr. Robert Kapp, a genetic toxicologist at Hazleton Laboratories who headed the chromosome investigation of DBCP workers, thinks that "we should look at the double Ys as being a possible barometer of what else is going on." He points out that a similar increase in doubling, or nondisjunction, of the twenty-first chromosome would increase a man's prospect of fathering a Down's baby.

More perhaps than any other environmental incident, DBCP set the scientific world to thinking about ways to ferret out chemicals whose prolonged general use may mean, if not mass sterility, at the least that a lot of people wake up one day to find they cannot have children at all. These thoughts have again and again come back to one place and one concept: workplace monitoring. Even before DBCP, it was evident that the workplace in itself could be a reproductive hazard. The clubfooted children of the helicopter pilots, birth defects among the children of female anesthetists, and the high miscarriage rate of the wives of vinyl-chloride workers were all testimony to this point.

After Lathrop, however, it was more than evident that, in a society that often declines to properly use animal evidence to establish appropriate safety margins, the workplace commends itself as does no other environment to settling a lot of arguments about the true human damage from chemicals. Reproductive health is almost a unique endpoint for measuring and monitoring. By the time the "body count" of other diseases, such as cancer, kidney damage, or lung disease, manifests itself among workers— or, for that matter, the general population—years have usually gone by and it is too late to guard other people from harmful exposures. But, with reproductive health, contact with the chemical deluge tends to produce signs of trouble rather quickly. Low sperm counts among men, miscarriages among working women or women whose husbands work in close contact with toxins, and the appearance of birth defects in children of either male or female workers, all may become obvious in a matter of months. "Like it or not," Dr. Frank Lundin, head of the epidemiological branch of the Bureau of Radiological Health once briskly summarized this point, "selected populations have now been exposed to certain agents for years and they can tell us a lot about what this may mean for the rest of us."

Actually, like it or not, selected populations—meaning, essentially, the industrial workforce—are probably destined to sustain relatively intense toxic exposures as long as society produces chemicals and industrial products. The 1970 Occupational Safety and Health Act guarantees that "insofar as [is] practicable, no employee will suffer diminished health, functional capacity or life expectancy as a result of his work experience," but for various reasons, both federal law and industrial custom still allow for workplace exposures that even the most callous observers would think intolerable should the population at large be routinely exposed to them. These reasons include the intense lobbying against workplace health now common in industry, accompanied by often quite exaggerated claims of the expense involved in improving workplace conditions, and they include the prevailing reality that American industry can choose to escape all regulation by fleeing to countries that haven't the least intent of controlling occupational exposures within their own borders. The American asbestos textile industry, for example, has now all but fully relocated to Mexico, Taiwan, Spain, and Brazil—a relocation that, unfortunately, various American tax and tariff regulations actually encourage. In a recent report to the Congressional Office of Technological Assessment, Barry Castleman, a Washington-based environmental consultant, suggested that American jobs be protected against this easy and cynical fleeing by, among other measures, raising tariffs to reflect the costs of pollution control and worker safety that American multinational companies avoid by moving their manufacturing operations elsewhere.

In any case, striking differentials between public and workplace exposures are now commonplace. It is, for instance, the position of the Nuclear Regulatory Commission that workers in atomic energy plants may receive up to five rads a year of radiation; but the stated goal of the government is that the general public should encounter only five rads of radiation from "all sources other than medical" every thirty years—this lower radiation exposure being one, it may be recalled, that some critics believe could in itself raise the American cancer rate by 10 percent over the years. Or, again, there is lead. In 1978, the Environmental Protection Agency issued its first national standard for lead in air of 1.5 micrograms per cubic meter; but the most recent proposal from the National Institute of Occupational Safety and Health (NIOSH) for workplace exposures to lead is 50 micrograms per cubic meter. In the general atmosphere, this higher exposure would be calamitous, probably causing an epidemic of childhood brain damage such as has never before been seen.

Irony holds much sway over human life, and there is a bitter irony in these higher workplace exposures. In a sense, the worse conditions are for workers, the better the workplace functions for the rest of us as a harbinger of chemicals that may generally threaten reproduction and that, like DBCP, the government will eventually decide are too dangerous for anyone to contact. Reproduction is rather a quixotic function; while at high toxic exposures it may present one of the first measurable signs of bodily distress, at lower exposures, the destruction of the ability to reproduce can be a long-term and insidious business. A 1971 experiment of Dr. Henry Schroeder, then a professor of physiology at Dartmouth Medical College, gives some idea of the potential for reproduction to fall away in silence, destroyed without other signs of warning. Dr. Schroeder thought to add very low levels of trace elements—including arsenic, lead, selenium, nickel, and cadmium—to the drinking water of mice and rats. The levels added, which ranged from three parts per million for selenium to twenty-five ppm for lead, did "not affect the rates of growth of mice or rats as compared to controls [or] affect reasonably long-term survival or cause early mortality [or], except in the case of lead . . . affect longevity." Yet these low levels of trace elements were the deathblow to reproduction. After two or three generations, the mice given lead, selenium, and cadmium simply died out. Although some could still manage to mate and conceive, the young they did conceive were stillborn or runts who died early.

✻

For various reasons, little attempt has been made to reap the particular lessons the workplace has to offer. This is partly due to what the government wants to study. The government, not unlike the rest of us, is obsessed with cancer, and the great bulk of what it spends to monitor health in industry goes toward compiling the cancer rates of workers; the National Institute of Occupational Safety and Health, the research arm of OSHA—the Occupational Safety and Health Administration—spends little time or money investigating birth defects among their children. In human terms, Joseph K. Wagoner, past president of the Society for Occupational and Environmental Health, is among those who consider this preoccupation "grossly misplaced." To Dr. Wagoner, it is "of course sad when people die of cancer ten years before they should. But it is tragic when a whole life is blighted by a birth defect and our research emphasis does not reflect this."

The situation is also partly due to what industry will permit to be studied. From a legal standpoint, workers who are part of state workers' compensation programs to some extent surrender their individual right to sue over job injuries, but they cannot surrender the right of their children to sue for birth defects. Industry, not surprisingly, tends to fight hardest against monitoring projects that focus on reproductive trouble. "Every company in the country," a chemical industry lawyer conceded a few years ago in the *New York Times,* "would be terrified about the prospect of having a deformed child bring suit against it."

Between these forces, the government has come to know very little about the fertility of workers and the health of those children they do have. Pregnancy problems, for example, are not a mandated "reportable condition" for the logs of workplace injuries and illnesses that industries engaged in interstate commerce now must maintain for periodic review by the Labor Department; the first National Natality Survey that actually asked new mothers and fathers about hazardous exposures in their occupational environment was not undertaken until 1978—and will not be compiled for years. And, except for two highly persistent women—Clara Schiffer, a program analyst in the office of the Secretary of HEW, and Vilma Hunt, an associate professor of Environmental Health at Pennsylvania State University—the government would barely have gotten as far as it has.

Hunt and Schiffer had become particularly concerned about the health of women who stayed on their jobs while they were pregnant. With Schiffer basically corraling the funds and Hunt the research, they produced in 1975 a 123-page report to the Secretary of HEW titled "Occupational Health Problems of Pregnant Women." This report put between two covers much of the available knowledge and research—essential parts of it from East European and Soviet studies—about the hazards to pregnancy associated with various working conditions, a compendium that had not previously existed in the United States. One leading government health official described reading "Occupational Health Problems of Pregnant Women," with its dry, relentless account of pathological pregnancies among operating-room personnel, toxicosis of pregnancy among women workers in DDT production, and premature labor in superphosphate factories, as being "a bit like when St. Paul was on the road to Damascus and the scales fell from his eyes."

For an HEW publication, "Occupational Health Problems of Pregnant Women" was a best seller, a compendium read widely in government and one that opened many eyes not just to pregnancy problems, but to the whole matter of reproductive health. Apparently, however, the scales have yet to fall quite far enough from either government or industry eyes. If DBCP is the agent that, in the past few years, has been confirmed as perhaps representing the most serious and widespread threat to male fertility, the herbicide 2,4,5-T represents the general contaminant that probably has most seriously threatened women's ability to carry to term the children they do conceive. It is, of course, a commonplace for industry today to bitterly complain of being overmonitored and overregulated. Yet, for all the complaints and the general impression that "very toxic" substances are now well controlled, it remained for six men in California to force DBCP to public attention; similarly, it remained for eight women in Oregon to force the issue on 2,4,5-T.

In counterpoint to DBCP, which had somehow managed to remain so anonymous that not even the Oil, Chemical and Atomic Workers were particularly aware of its toxicity, 2,4,5-T has long been one of the most scrutinized and bitterly condemned environmental contaminants. Developed by the American military during post–World War II research into biological warfare, its first real notoriety came in the 1960s when, as an ingredient in Agent Orange and other herbicides, it was used to defoliate thousands of acres of Vietnamese jungle. When the Army started this defoliation program, no one seems to have tested 2,4,5-T on a single mouse. By the mid-1960s, however, it had been demonstrated that 2,4,5-T is a very potent teratogen in animals, its major impact on the fetus stemming from dioxin, or TCDD, an inevitable contaminant of 2,4,5-T production. The worries about possible birth defects to human children were a major, if officially unacknowledged, reason for the defoliation program's being halted in 1970.

A decade later, however, 2,4,5-T, which is hardly the sort of thing that disappears on cue, remains an inexorable presence in Vietnam. John Pilger, an English journalist, has described its poisonous footprints in a 1979 article on the Op-Ed page of the *New York Times*. He wrote:

I went back to Vietnam last year. Much of the North, which few Americans ever saw, is a moonscape. All visible signs of life—houses, factories, pagodas, churches—have been oblit-

erated. Forty-four percent of the forests have been destroyed; in many of those still standing, there are no longer
birds and animals. There are thousands of children in Hanoi
and Haiphong alone who are permanently deaf as a result of
the bombing at Christmas 1972. . . . There are deformed
infants, damaged in the womb as a result of the poisoning of
the landscape.

Some people think it possible that Americans exposed to
2,4,5-T in Vietnam brought home its apparent ability to deform
with them. There are widespread reports, among them a recent
informal *New York Times* investigation, that men in close contact
with 2,4,5-T father unusual numbers of deformed children. The
*Times* investigated the health of eighteen veterans and civilians
who had worked with 2,4,5-T. Thirteen of these men were
married. Only two couples among them had normal children. One
couple was childless and the other ten had had a total of five
deformed children and eight stillborn children. While these numbers are, needless to say, suggestive of trouble, such informal reports have yet to be confirmed by a proper, random epidemiological survey.

The more substantial reason to worry about 2,4,5-T in the
United States is that, until 1979, when the EPA evoked its
emergency ban, more 2,4,5-T–containing defoliants, with their
noxious dioxin contaminant, were being used domestically than
had ever been flung at Vietnam. The Vietnamese defoliation
program lasted from 1962 to 1970. During that time, about five
million total acres of jungle and countryside were sprayed; in the
United States over the past decade, about five million acres of
forests, pastures, and rangeland have been sprayed with 2,4,5-T–
containing defoliants *every year;* and the government itself, in the
form of the Agriculture Department and Forest Service, has been
its chief user. These agencies employ 2,4,5-T to kill weeds, clear
land, and thin forests of unwanted trees.

What particularly stands out about the domestic use of 2,4,5-
T is that no adverse evidence seemed strong enough to end the

government's endorsement of it. Scientists showed that rhesus monkeys fed a diet containing just 500 parts per trillion (a trillion is a million times a million, or a thousand billions) of the herbicide's dioxin contaminant began to die within seven months; they showed that mice fed just 5 ppt dioxin developed unusual numbers of tumors. Many biologists are now in agreement with Dr. Matthew Meselson, a Harvard University biochemistry professor, who has since described dioxin as "the most powerful small molecule known and, it is beginning to appear, the most powerful carcinogen known."

Environmental groups, and just plain citizens hoping to keep out of the path of aerial spraying, who had sued the government almost nonstop for a decade, invariably failed in the courts. The Dow Chemical Company, the chief American manufacturer of 2,4,5-T, countered that the "trace levels" of dioxin left when the sprays were properly used were harmless—a position that it was able to uphold in court and in various skirmishes at the EPA, until the incident of the Oregon miscarriages. After the eight Oregon women complained of having lost their babies soon after 2,4,5-T spraying near their homes, the EPA commissioned the Environmental Health Institute of Colorado State University and the University of Miami Medical School to study miscarriage rates in Alsea, Oregon. Although this study is widely felt to have suffered somewhat in design because of the haste to get it completed before the next spring's spraying, it did find that, in June, or about a month after the spraying, the rate of reported miscarriage in Alsea for the previous six years had averaged 130 per 1000 live births; by contrast, the miscarriage rate in both the urban areas of Eugene and Corvallis and in an unsprayed rural area were about 45 per 1000 live births.

According to the EPA, in the years preceding 1979, the 2,4,5-T spraying of forests, pasturelands, and powerline rights-of-way had annually exposed four million people, including pregnant women, to dioxin. Moreover, even the EPA's emergency "ban" of 2,4,5-T only applied to the spraying of forests, pastures, and powerline rights-of-way. Two other major uses—spraying rice fields and rangeland—are still permitted. The EPA has said that few people are in the direct path of such spraying; however, since dioxin appears to build up in the food chain, people don't have to contact it directly to get a dose. Up to 60 ppt of dioxin, or twelve times the concentration known to cause tumors in mice, has been detected in the fatty tissue of cattle that have grazed on 2,4,5-T–treated rangeland. A preliminary sampling of twenty-five nursing mothers in four states has also confirmed the presence of from 10 to 41 ppt dioxin in the breast milk of residents of Oregon and Texas.*

Clearly, 2,4,5-T is a very special case in the annals of environmentalism. This was not an instance where people were proceeding against a few animal experiments and mild questions. By any reasoned standard, the evidence against 2,4,5-T was overwhelming years ago—and it included human evidence to back up the animal observations. The particular problem 2,4,5-T illustrates is that "reasonable" or even "overwhelming" evidence is sometimes not enough in environmental cases. Because industries have political influence, because judges don't understand biology, because it is hard for people to accept that a mistake of the magnitude of 2,4,5-T could be made, evidence in environmental cases sometimes has to be dramatically and spectacularly overwhelming before it is accepted. The workplace provided such evidence against DBCP; could it also have readily provided evidence of dioxin's impact on pregnancy years earlier?

In the case of dioxin, it is not easy to say. The most dramatic evidence against this "most powerful small molecule" has actually come from the workplace—but it is also evidence that has been severely challenged. The answer revolves around the possible

---

* Although its identification in breast milk shows how far up the food chain a toxin has insinuated itself, except, perhaps, where there may have been very severe and unusual local pollution episodes, such identification is not reason for mothers to give up breast-feeding. Virtually all widespread environmental contaminants, such as pesticides and herbicides, found in human milk are also found in the cow's milk that forms the basis of most commercial formulas. On the other hand, human milk is saved some contamination simply because it doesn't go through an assembly line; its lead content, for example, is negligible by comparison with the lead found in many formulas.

impact on pregnancy of hexachlorophene-containing disinfectant soaps. Such soaps, which are partly formulated from a precursor of 2,4,5-T, are also inevitably contaminated with dioxin during their manufacture. In the early 1970s, the Givaudan Corporation, a Swiss company that is the world's largest manufacturer of hexachlorophene, publicly conceded that its "pure hexachlorophene" was contaminated with 20 ppb of dioxin—a level said to have since been lowered to 10 ppb. Many people may recall encountering hexachlorophene in a variety of consumer products, which once ranged from anti-acne soaps to vaginal sprays. By the 1960s, it had also become so routine in hospitals to wash newborns with a hexachlorophene solution that, in the phrase of journalist Thomas Whiteside, an obdurate chronicler of dioxin, "the stuff seemed to serve almost as a sort of sheep-dip in hospital nurseries."

The consumer use of hexachlorophene came to an end in the United States and in several other nations in the early 1970s when it was realized that some premature babies had sustained fatal brain lesions from their hexachlorophene baths. In the worst such incidents, forty French infants died in 1972 after being dusted with talcum powder that had been mistakenly mixed with 6 percent hexachlorophene. Nonetheless, hospitals continue to be the work environment that, aside from crop spraying, would seem to involve the most intense exposures to dioxin. Even in those nations where the general consumer use of hexachlorophene products has been banned, they remain in lavish, and quite legal, use in hospitals and other health facilities.

In this capacity, hexachlorophene soaps now stand accused of causing severe birth defects to the children of nurses who contact them during pregnancy. Since hexachlorophene easily penetrates the skin and migrates rapidly into the blood, it would not be surprising that it, and its dioxin contaminant, could reach the fetus in teratogenic doses. Dr. Hildegard Halling, the chief physician of the Department of Chronic Somatic Diseases at Södertälje Hospital near Stockholm, Sweden, raised this issue in 1978 when she told a conference at the New York Academy of Sciences about her retrospective study of children born to nurses who had typically washed their hands in hexachlorophene soaps from ten to sixty-three times a day. As reported by Dr. Halling, the rate of birth defects among their children was as devastating as any ever seen in a workplace setting. Twenty-five of the 460 children born to these nurses had severe defects, which embraced a range of their bodily systems, including the heart, lungs, and central nervous system. Another 46 children had minor abnormalities.

There are, however, statistical problems with the Halling study. Basically, she did not take a random sample of women exposed to hexachlorophene, but studied hexachlorophene use among women at three hospitals that had recently experienced unusual birth-defect "clusters." As such clusters may be just an expression of chance, the study design does not prove that hexachlorophene is at fault. In a March 1979 letter to the *New England Journal of Medicine,* the Swedish National Board of Health said that, after reviewing more than 4500 pregnancies of hospital workers, it had found no difference between the perinatal deaths or malformation rates of children born to women who had worked in hospitals where there was "extensive use of hexachlorophene" and those who worked in hospitals where "hexachlorophene was not used at all or only sporadically." Neither, however, are these preliminary observations from the Swedish Board of Health an acquittal. The full study has yet to be published and it is not yet evident—among other things—whether the board's "extensive users" washed their hands in hexachlorophene as often as did the women Halling studied.

The standoff concerning severe defects does not, however, detract from concern about the possibly more subtle impact of an agent like dioxin. The substantial evidence of excess miscarriages among 2,4,5-T–exposed women certainly suggests that, if dioxin is not also causing severe defects, it may at least be harming the fetus in other ways. The whole trend of prenatal research, after all, has been to show that agents that cause miscarriages in early pregnancy may well leave behind surviving fetuses who have sustained injuries ranging from latent cancer to neurological deficits. "For example," Thomas Whiteside has asked in the *New Yorker,* "who could pinpoint a cause-and-effect relationship involving dioxin if a child of a dioxin-exposed mother should turn out to be just a little bit less alert than the average, a little more prone to memory lapses, a little more 'nervous,' or a little more susceptible to diseases of various kinds?"

Given the extent to which exposure to hexachlorophene may involve the unborn children of female hospital personnel in such risks, Dr. Carl Keller of the epidemiology branch of the National Institute of Child Health and Human Development wonders why people even bother to further ponder or research the matter. Dr. Keller points out that there are plenty of other disinfectant agents. "When you have a substance you know is this toxic and you know it is absorbable, why mess with it in this way?" he asks. As for the extent to which dioxin has contaminated the general environment, some observations from Dr. James Van Allen, a pathologist at the University of Wisconsin Primate Research Center, are pertinent. Dr. Allen has shown a consistent genius for ferreting out truly dangerous substances and testing them on monkeys—which is the closest science can get to human experimentation—at levels humans may be commonly encountering in their own environment. Not long ago, Dr. Allen fed eight female rhesus monkeys a diet containing 50 ppt dioxin—an amount, of course, now to be found in the fatty tissue of some American meat. After seven months, these females were mated. Two did not conceive at all despite repeated matings. Four who did conceive had spontaneous abortions. Only two managed to conceive and carry an infant to term.

If DBCP and dioxin have, in varying degrees, suggested the potential of workplace studies for protecting the fetus—and protecting people's very chances of having children—it is not so clear how the government, or anyone else, can go about gathering information about reproduction and occupation. Since many women still live with the fear that a pregnancy will see them fired from their jobs, they often elect to conceal their condition for as long as possible. As for men, Dr. Donald Whorton, a San Francisco physician who has worked with the Oil, Chemical and Atomic Workers on environmental health issues, including DBCP, does not think that going around to factories and taking sperm counts will ever be accepted as a routine practice. He points out that the Lathrop situation was unique. "There was a stable work force. The men knew each other and there was social interaction among their wives and they all really figured this out for themselves. No one told them to get a count taken. On the other hand, even in other situations where there is good reason to suspect trouble, you may have trouble getting cooperation. People have religious objections since masturbation is involved. Men who are impotent won't cooperate because they don't want anyone to know. People are also afraid to find out what's happening to them. In Lathrop, there was one guy who wouldn't have a count because he said, 'What if I am really sterile and I know? No woman would want to marry me.' So, I think the best you can do is look for those situations where there is reasonably good animal evidence or other reasons to suspect something wrong. Then it's reasonable to ask people to cooperate. Taking everybody's sperm count all the time would probably cause a mass revolt."

From another point of view, Dr. Channing Meyer, the former chief of the medical section of NIOSH's Hazard Evaluation Branch and a great student of sperm, thinks that the scenario of the future holds such potential threats to reproduction that people will overcome their discomfiture to protect themselves. He emphasizes that sperm testing may be a better and quicker method of catching incipient industrial disease than even the blood and urine testing now required in some industries. "The sperm maturation process," he explains, "is one of the most rapidly dividing cell systems in the adult body and toxic agents have their greatest effect on rapidly dividing cells. The lining of the gastrointestinal tract and the bone-marrow production of blood cells are also fast-dividing systems, but obviously, they are hard to get at. Sperm are accessible, cheap, and a count is easy to make."

Interestingly, Dr. Meyer feels that perhaps the end of the industrial process—in the form of toxic wastes—may prove more threatening than the beginning of it in the form of toxic ingredients. "In virtually every part of the country," he points out, "we have so-called 'sanitary landfills'—meaning chemical dumps like Love Canal. Over the next ten to fifteen years as the containers in these dumps break down, there could be incredible contamination of the food and water supply. Who knows for sure? Very little could happen, or the result could be utter catastrophe. Personally, I am very concerned that we are going to modify our capacity to reproduce. Ultimately, it's going to smack the public in the face and they'll have to decide what they want done."

Some observers actually wonder whether there has already been some "modification" in the general ability to reproduce. In 1951, for example, Dr. John MacLeod, now a professor emeritus at Cornell University Medical College and probably the world's leading sperm expert, found the mean count in a sample of 1000 men to be 107 million per milliliter of ejaculate. Based largely on his work, a count of around 100 million or so has long been accepted as the American standard.

In recent years, however, the mean sperm counts of groups of men measured in populations in as diverse parts of the nation as Iowa and Texas have ranged between 50 and 80 million per milliliter of ejaculate. These more recent counts would seem to suggest a noteworthy general decrease in sperm production. Yet, back in New York, Dr. MacLeod examined another 9000 men between 1966 and 1976 and found their mean count to be 95 million—quite acceptable considering that most of them had come to him for suspected fertility problems. Can the counts elsewhere be explained? At one point, since all the recent counts except MacLeod's came from men awaiting vasectomies, it was suggested that nervousness had prompted a temporary plunge in their counts. But, having recently learned that the average count in a group of French men awaiting vasectomies was around 100 million, Dr. MacLeod does not accept the nerves explanation. Nor, for that matter, does he accept "some of these really low counts" as accurate. He thinks that the general sperm count "has been remarkably consistent over the years." Considering, however, the nature of some environmental toxins, Dr. MacLeod is "not ruling out the idea that there may be trouble in some areas of the country where maybe the water has been contaminated or something else has occurred to lower sperm counts locally."

Whether or not there has been a general lowering in the number or quality of sperm, there are clearly several special populations with demonstrated sperm impairment. The DES sons, with their all-around "pathological sperm"—among those affected, count, shape, and motility alike were abnormal—represent some thousands of young men. In industry, men who work with microwaves, lead, and chloroprene (a substance used in the manufacture of synthetic rubber) have all recently been found to have low sperm counts and sometimes abnormal sperm. The wives of chloroprene workers also appear to have about a threefold excess of miscarriage, certainly an indication that their husbands' sperm might have sustained lethal mutations. (When researchers think to ask the question, environmental agents associated with low sperm counts also tend to be associated with a "loss of libido" or sex drive—a comment, perhaps, on possible causes of impotence, a condition said to be much on the increase in the United States.)

Obviously, by now, these special populations add up to substantial numbers of people; it would hardly seem necessary to wait for a proven general decrease in the sperm count to start worrying about the impact of gonadotoxic agents.

The new interest in reproductive health in the workplace has had a bitter edge for many observers. Already it is the new "scientific" excuse to discriminate against *women* workers, especially those trying to move into some higher-paying blue collar and factory jobs. In 1976, for instance, both General Motors and Du Pont decided to forbid women any production jobs that involved exposures to lead. The practical effect of this decision, which a General Motors spokesman once explained had been made solely on "humanitarian grounds," was to bar the entire sex from these jobs on the grounds of pregnancies that had not even occurred yet—and may never occur. At present, most women seeking factory jobs appear to have already had the children they want.

The Du Pont and General Motors dictums, moreover, came right in the wake of research that had seriously indicted lead's impact on male reproduction. In 1975, for example, a group at the Institute for Scientific Research in New Mexico exposed both male and female animals to lead before mating them; it took the offspring of an unexposed control group about 66 seconds to learn to work their way out of a swimming maze, the offspring of lead-exposed fathers about 89 seconds to learn the same task, and the offspring of lead-exposed mothers about 92 seconds—the difference between exposing mothers and fathers obviously being negligible. Also in 1975, in a much-discussed report, the Rumanians said they had found unusually large numbers of abnormal sperm among workers in a lead-battery factory. The lead exposures of most of these men seemed to be well below the present official limit for industrial exposures in the United States. But, to Vilma Hunt, even after years of interest in reproductive health and all the meetings and conferences on the subject she has attended, it still remains "a wonder how often you have to remind men that they do actually produce sperm. In reproduction you are really talking about a triad of concerns—the egg, the sperm, and the fetus—all of which can be injured. You'd think, if nothing else, the revelation of sterility among DBCP workers would have enforced this point. But it hasn't entirely; and we're going to have to work very hard to make sure the components of the triad receive full and equal attention."

Aside, however, from being one of the shoddiest uses to which "science" has yet been put, this idea that reproductive health consists of keeping women out of factories is very dangerous in its error. The importance of the male contribution to reproductive health has been discussed; equally important, women would appear to require "protection" less from the higher-paying jobs they are seeking than from the lower-paying jobs they already have. Much traditional "women's work" involves rather extraordinary exposures to reproductive hazards. If, for example, American industry and society were really worried about "the unborn child," they would be very worried about the exposures to alkylating agents—a class of compounds that, in laboratory animals, appears to come in second only to the nitroso compounds in its potency as transplacental carcinogens—that the low-paid women in the textile and dry-cleaning industries often sustain. If people are really worried about the unborn child, they would worry that dental assistants—an employment category that is almost the exclusive turf of young women in the prime childbearing years—absorb about 50 percent more mercury in the course of preparing dental fillings than dentists do in the course of caulking the prepared mixture into cavities. And people would also be worried about the American housewife, a person who, in a day that may take her from polishing furniture to cleaning ovens, deals with more toxins than do many professional chemists. When, for example, vinyl chloride was still used as an aerosol propellant, a woman spraying her hair in a closed bathroom would have absorbed more of the stuff than would a worker at any of Dow's American plants in an eight-hour day.

A really good place, however, for everyone to start their worrying about this subject would be the health industry itself. It is hard to think of any other work environment that presents a more intense mélange of known hazards to the fetus than hospitals; they are not only strewn with chemicals, anesthetic gases, radiation equipment, and sonar machines, but they are also a gathering place for sick people who may be carriers of any number of biological organisms—the rubella, mumps, herpes, and influenza viruses, the typhoid bacillus, syphilis spirochete, and malaria protozoa, to name but some—known to injure the fetus. It is also hard to think of another working environment as systematically organized, not just to put women in low-paying positions, but to put them in the positions that involve the most intense hazardous exposures.

Radiologists, for example, have tended to congratulate themselves because their death rate—which in past decades was high not only for cancer, but for a number of other diseases—is now pretty much in line with that of other physician specialists. The improvement in the health of radiologists has paralleled some improvements in radiation protection; but it has also paralleled a great change in employment practices in radiology. Radiologists themselves now usually limit their role to interpreting X-ray pictures; technologists, most of whom are young and female, are now likely to be the people who actually *take* X-ray pictures. As of 1970, 45,000 women in the prime child-bearing years of sixteen to thirty-four were employed as radiation technologists. No one has ever systematically studied their health—or, indeed, the health of their children; yet, in the past twenty years, the Bureau of Radiological Health, the National Cancer Institute, and National Institutes of Health have sponsored almost constant investigations of the health of male radiologists.

In the laboratory, the setting is about the same. Medical technologists are the people who work in hospital laboratories, doing tests, mixing drugs, identifying viruses, and inhaling chemical fumes. In 1973, the American Society of Clinical Pathologists estimated that 85 to 90 percent of them were female. A year later, NIOSH published a survey of health practices in some five thousand hospitals. Fewer than half these institutions had in-service training to instruct their personnel in safe ways to approach radiation, chemicals, infectious disease, and other dangers; and, among those with in-service training, fewer than 2 percent placed any emphasis on special precautions to be taken during pregnancy. Actually, not even so clear-cut a hazard as the high rate of miscarriage and malformed children seen among operating-room personnel seems to have moved all hospitals to act. In 1974, the journal *Anesthesiology* had editorialized that "in the light of present knowledge" about the birth defects and other harms attributed to anesthesia, "failure to install exhaust systems (in all areas in which inhalation anesthetics are administered) and failure to use them at all times represents an unconscionable practice." But, by 1976, only half the nation's operating rooms had been equipped with scavenging devices; and only in 1978 did OSHA issue a standard that would require all of them to be so equipped.

Under these circumstances, the results of some recent surveys of pregnancy outcome among female hospital personnel are not surprising. A 1978 preliminary report on birth defects and employment from the Center for Disease Control, for example, while heavily qualified by the small number of people sampled at that time, did suggest that "female health workers" had the highest birth defect rate of any employment category investigated; by contrast, male health workers, most of whom would presumably be physicians, did not father an unusual number of malformed youngsters. As part of its hexachlorophene research, the Swedish National Board of Health has also reported that, on the whole, female hospital workers give birth to more malformed children than usually expected in Sweden. Based on the available evidence, a good argument might be made that the health profession itself could unilaterally make a nice dent in the incidence of birth defects by encouraging women to become the people who supervise and write prescriptions and read X-ray plates from a healthy distance—while men become the people who empty bedpans, take blood, snap X-ray pictures, wash their hands constantly in hexachlorophene, and do laboratory work.

To point out that sperm and eggs seem to stand fairly equal before toxins and that men and women should stand absolutely equal in opportunities for employment is not to deny that the situation changes after conception. There is no argument that, once she is pregnant, a woman does have, in the phrase of a feminist health commentator, "a unique employment problem." That problem is that, even leaving aside intense toxic exposures and major birth defects, quite low exposure to many sorts of chemicals may subtly damage an unborn child. Anesthesia is an example. In 1978, the Occupational Safety and Health Administration, as its first standard ever promulgated for operating rooms, decided to require that background levels of anesthesia in the air of these places not exceed 10 ppm.

While somewhat higher than the 2 ppm that NIOSH had originally suggested, the 10 ppm standard was a clear improvement over the background levels of 100 ppm or more often found in unscavenged operating rooms. But was it low enough to protect the fetus? In 1974, Dr. Kelvin L. Quimby, a University of Wisconsin psychologist, had exposed one group of rats to 10 ppm of halothane, a commonly used anesthetic, during their prenatal life, and given another group the same treatment after they were sixty days old. In later life, the rats prenatally exposed to the 10 ppm of halothane for several days made 30 percent more errors in working their way through a maze than did the rats exposed as sixty-day-old adults. Brain autopsies of the prenatally exposed animals showed that they had sustained a "permanent failure of formation of the synaptic web and postsynaptic membranes in 30 percent of the postsynaptic membranes," while the adult rats had only sustained "slight neuronal damage." Quimby and his co-workers wondered "whether or not pregnant women should avoid chronic halothane exposure even at trace levels of 10 ppm as a precaution against enduring damage to the brain of the fetus." Presumably, the same question applies to scores of chemical substances.

*

The final irony is that occupation and reproductive health may not, in the end, be that complex an issue. Of course, workplace health is no simple matter; it involves, in the summary of one commentator, "our economic and social structure, our labor agreements, the physical design of plants, equipment, work methods, product quality, hours of work, selection and training of workers—including sex and nationality." Within all this complexity, however, the unvarnished goal of trying to protect people during the relatively short period of time that most Western humans devote to reproducing stands out as much simpler—as being a time when various public policies and brief cooperation between employers and employees could bestow a lifetime's benefit on a child. The Soviet Union, many East European countries, and some Western European ones have, for example, adapted an obvious solution to the "unique employment problem" of pregnant women; they simply transfer these women, without loss of pay or seniority, to nonhazardous jobs for the duration of their pregnancies.

The Dow Chemical Company, rather oddly, has supplied about as good evidence as there is that reproduction and industry are not drastically incompatible pursuits. This company has fought government regulation at every turn; through products such as 2,4,5-T and DBCP, it has thrown giant, dark shadows over the reproductive health of the general population. It seems a great waste that Dow Chemical—and other companies—so frantically commit themselves to chemicals with so sincerely frightening a potential for mass harm when there is good evidence that the industrial societies can function quite well without them. The animal laboratory, after all, has suggested that the percentage of carcinogens among all chemicals is relatively so small that industrial societies need not depend on such substances; if, further, there is a human laboratory for reproductive health, Dow headquarters is quite possibly it.

Midland, Michigan, is where, in the 1890s, Herbert Dow began experimenting with various chemical processes and where the Dow Chemical Company still maintains both its world headquarters and "the largest chemical plant in the world within one fence line." The Dow Midland complex produces more than 530 chemical, plastic, and agricultural products, employs more than 6,400 people, and includes more than thirty laboratories devoted to research and development. Altogether, despite some ingenuous local efforts to overlook the fact—the Chamber of Commerce likes to refer to Midland as "the city of beautiful churches"— Midland city and county are headquarters to a chemical intensity matched in very few places on the globe; yet the local birth-defects rate, as reflected in county figures, is unremarkable.

From 1961 through 1978, the latest year available, the birth-defects rate in Midland County was often lower than in the rest of Michigan, and rarely more than a few tenths of a percentage point above it. The exception occurred from 1971 to 1974 when the Midland rate abruptly doubled, and then tripled, before plunging downward again. These four years of high defects could have been a random variation; they could, of course, also reflect that something went awry at Dow or at another company in the area; but there is something intriguing about the Midland excess during those years. Most of the excess consisted of heart defects, limb defects, and undescended testes. These defects have all been to a greater or lesser extent associated with hormone supports. It would not be surprising to learn that some scatterbrained obstetrician in Midland, as did scatterbrained obstetricians throughout the country in the early 1970s, went on a binge of prescribing hormones to pregnant patients.

That the Midland birth-defects rate has generally been unremarkable does not, of course, mean that children in the city and county may not have sustained more subtle damage; it certainly does not say what is happening to reproduction near whatever places Dow disposes of the chemical wastes generated by "the largest chemical plant in the world within one fence line." And it does not mean that Dow is totally free of health problems. When tested in 1977, for example, 33 percent of the DBCP-exposed workers at Dow's Magnolia, Arkansas, plant had a sperm count of 0. By comparison, "only" 2 percent of DBCP-exposed workers at the Shell Chemical Company's Mobile, Alabama, plant and 7 percent of those at Shell's Denver, Colorado, plant had counts of 0.

Still, if the price for "progress" in Midland seems not to have been a trail of pathological sperm, miscarriages, and children who are missing obvious parts of their bodies and brains, why should it be the price anywhere?

For industrial countries, the population-per-obstetrician ratio, and the population-per-pediatrician ratio unexpectedly significantly relate in a negative way to the infant mortality rate. The population-per-nurse and the nurse-and-midwife ratios are, interestingly, positively related to the infant mortality rate. It is not clear what these statistical relationships mean, but they offer little support for the importance of medical care as distributed by physicians in reducing infant mortality.

IRVIN EMANUEL, M.D.
in *Birth Defects: Risks and Consequences*

# Chapter 8

# HEALTH AT BIRTH AND AT LARGE

In June 1973, at Brown Lakes, Wisconsin, the American Academy of Pediatrics, in cooperation with some HEW agencies, held its first full-scale conference on the subject of environmental threats to the young. That such a conference was held at all represented a turning point in the disease perceptions of physicians; and, when published a year later as a special supplement to *Pediatrics,* the papers from the conference, which had covered topics ranging from "The Placental Transmission of Chemicals in the Subhuman

Primate" to the "Effects of Air Pollution on Children," provided a valuable commentary on the environmental health concerns of this age group. They also, however, provided a graphic if unwitting comment on a certain medical myopia. None of the doctors who authored these twenty-three papers had thought to focus on the idea that the hospital itself is the first environment that most Western children encounter, and that newborns, a population at severe risk for environmental stress, have become a population on which medicine has focused an extraordinary technological arsenal.

The American hospital today is a place where children are often pushed into labor by potent hormones; where they face double the chance of being brought into the world by a caesarean operation that they did even five years ago, where the plastics that leach from the bags holding intravenous solutions and blood are thought to perhaps contribute to necrotizing enterocolitis, a degenerative and sometimes fatal disease of the intestines whose incidence among newborns has markedly increased in recent years; where the fetus is routinely exposed to anesthetics whose long-term effects are simply unknown; where careless inductions not infrequently contribute to respiratory distress; and where what Jane Brody, the *New York Times* health reporter, has described as the "Orwellian scene of electronically controlled childbirth" has become commonplace.

By "electronically controlled," Ms. Brody is referring to the fetal monitoring equipment that, in both external and internal versions, is increasingly used to check the status of the child during labor as a substitute for the "old-fashioned" method of checking the fetal heartbeat with a stethoscope. (In the external version, the mother wears a large "sonar belt"; in the internal, electrodes and wiring are inserted through her vagina to be attached to the fetal scalp.) Although fetal monitoring is widely conceded to be of use during "high-risk" deliveries, its routine use is a very controversial subject. The equipment is expensive, cumbersome for the mother, and, many feel, not fully reliable. The National Center for Health Services Research, an HEW agency, recently condemned routine fetal monitoring as the source of perhaps $400 million a year in unnecessary medical expenses—a large part of it in the form of caesareans mistakenly performed when the information from monitoring equipment was "misread" to indicate that the child was in immediate distress.

When *Pediatrics* did focus on the potential medical dangers to children during labor and birth, the journal turned to Great Britain for a commentator. The British have not lagged far behind Americans in their own medicalization of birth, but they have begun to have more searching second thoughts about what they are doing—at least on paper. (The amount of radiation involved in British births hardly suggests their obstetricians have made a great leap toward reform.) In any case, the September 1976 publication in *Pediatrics* of a "commentary" by Dr. Iain Chalmers of the Welsh National School of Medicine seems to have been the first overall critical appraisal of current obstetric practice to appear in a major American journal. "Development and innovation in the management of childbirth over the past ten years has taken place at a rate which is unparalleled," Dr. Chalmers commented. "Care during pregnancy has been extended and elaborated to include assessment of fetal well-being with placental function tests and serial ultrasound cephalometry. . . . Efficient pharmacological control of labor with oxytocin and prostaglandins has increased the scope for induction and augmentation of labor. . . . Policies of universal hospital confinement have been promoted, and, in many maternity units, the use of partography, cardiotocography, fetal blood sampling, and lumbar epidural block [an anesthetic technique] has become routine. In spite of the background of science against which many of these developments have been introduced, there have been few systematic attempts to evaluate their effects. Their relative importance in contributing to reduced perinatal and maternal mortality rates, if any, is not known."

Equally important, the "relative importance" of such techniques in actually contributing to the adverse outcome of pregnancy is also unknown. There are many gaps in medical research, but surely it stands out as a particularly large gap that only now are researchers beginning to really scrutinize the possible side effects of medical techniques and agents employed during the early, most delicate moments of life. For example, astounding as it may seem, considering that easily 90 percent of American infants are exposed to major obstetrical anesthesia, the first long-term study of the neurological effects of such anesthesia on the fetus is still being worked on; and even with the caesarean rate climbing yearly, there is still no substantial long-term follow-up of caesarean children.

Since World War II, both maternal deaths during childbirth and infant mortality rates have declined steadily in the Western world. In obstetrics, these lowered rates are sometimes seen as a certain justification for the past ten years of "unparalleled development and innovation." As have other commentators, however, Dr. Chalmers observes that events outside obstetrics actually account for a large part of the decline in maternal and infant deaths. Fifteen years ago, for example, the survival rate for infants who weighed less than 1000 grams (about 2.2 pounds) at birth was about 10 percent—no matter how well or badly an obstetrician brought them into the world. The equipment capable of helping them to breathe and function simply did not yet exist; but today, in a well-equipped center, the survival chances for these children reaches toward 50 percent. Mothers, meanwhile, are surviving birth better at least partly because of the biological bonuses of having fewer children.

There have, of course, also been obstetrical contributions to the lowered infant and maternal death rates. Contemporary obstetrics has decisively conquered the medieval horrors that once meant that pregnancy complications and death walked hand in hand; obstetricians have also become very adept at handling some types of difficult pregnancies—those of diabetic women are a chief example—where medical hovering, even to the point of hospitalizing the mother for a large part of the pregnancy, works to advantage. These are no small accomplishments; and yet some commentators wonder whether there has not been a price for them, in an increased hovering over all pregnancies, which is perhaps generally detrimental. Dr. Irvin Emanuel has pointed out that, in the industrialized world, higher obstetrician-per-population ratios tend to be associated not with lower, but with *higher* infant mortality rates. He goes on to remark that, while many complex factors are evidently involved in this disconcerting ratio, certainly it is a trend that invites consideration of the idea that, in its current aggressive form, Western obstetrics may provide "benefits to a small number of women with special problems [which are] counterbalanced by common practices to the many which are not beneficial."

Dr. Emanuel's comments bring to mind, of course, that only after DES was discovered to be a carcinogen did researchers carefully reevaluate the obstetric records of the "perfect population" at Chicago and finally show that it also seemed to have caused an immediate increase in early infant deaths. DES, in short, was one fairly "common practice to the many" whose fatal edge went unobserved for about thirty years. As other "innovative" obstetrical techniques and drugs receive the attention long overdue them, it seems likely that other unsettling news will follow.

Artificial induction of labor involves launching labor before it begins of its own accord, and usually includes the administration of a synthetic version of oxytocin, the hormone that naturally controls a woman's contractions during childbirth. There are, to be sure, medically valid reasons for induction; postmaturity, for example, can be a quite dangerous condition. Traditionally, however, most inductions in the United States have been "elective" procedures. Despite much editorializing against the practice, a large portion of them are done for "the social convenience" of either doctors or mothers who can't be bothered to wait for a baby to put in its own inconvenient late-night or weekend appearance; they also seem to be done simply as part of the medical fascination for "controlling" biological processes. As early as 1955, 5 percent of all live births in New York City were induced births. By the mid-1970s, many hospitals in England and the United States were inducing labor in 20 or 30 percent or even more of their patients—or, at least, their private patients. Since the social convenience of poorer women is not a particular medical concern, these women largely escaped the fad for induction.

Certain drawbacks to induced birth have long been obvious. The harder, quicker contractions brought on by the excess oxytocin escalate the mother's need for anesthesia and other drugs; inductions sometimes simply "fail" and must be completed as caesareans. And, since something might go wrong during induced births more quickly than it otherwise would, doctors almost invariably order X rays before inductions.

Still, close evaluation of induced birth was not forthcoming until a few years ago. Perhaps the single most condemnatory report on induced birth is a 1975 examination of the circumstances surrounding 100 consecutive cases of respiratory distress syndrome among infants born at Yale–New Haven Hospital, the teaching hospital of Yale Medical School. After going over the records of these children, a team of doctors concluded that fifteen respiratory distress cases—including three fatalities—had occurred because the physician induced birth without having appropriately tested for the gestational age of the fetus. Another eighteen cases, including one death, were said to have occurred when the physician, although having done appropriate tests, proceeded to induce without "adequate" reasons.

The substantial question surrounding this procedure, however, has been that of permanent deficits to the young. In 1975, in a searching look at the immediate aftermath of induction, the National Childbirth Trust of England found that induced infants were twice as likely to be delivered by forceps, had quadruple the chance of spending time in a "special care unit," and had double the number of breathing and sucking problems. (In the minds of some observers, sucking problems—meaning the child does not nurse well—are among the earliest signs of possible neurological damage.) Since there has yet to be any substantial long-term follow-up of the later social and educational adjustment of induced children, there is no way to say whether these immediate signs of distress did mark long-term deficits. In considering the prospects of permanent injury, however, one important thing to look at is the relationship between jaundice and induced birth.

Jaundice, a condition in which the bile pigment bilirubin builds up in the blood, body, and finally the brain, briefly strikes perhaps half of all newborn children. Except for special cases brought on by defined causes, such as blood disorders or liver malfunctions, these brief bouts of "newborn" or "physiological jaundice," as they are sometimes termed, usually pass without harm or the need for treatment as the child adjusts to postnatal life.

Still, newborn jaundice does make people nervous. For infants, even moderate bilirubin buildups carry the threat of permanent brain damage, which may manifest itself as mental retardation, psychological disturbances, hearing impairment, incoordination, and other symptoms. Yet, because exchange transfusion, the traditional treatment for jaundice, was itself a risky procedure for the newborn, doctors were reluctant to intervene. In the late 1960s, however, the discovery of phototherapy—in essence, bathing the infant in special, powerful lights—decidedly improved the terms of treatment. For reasons not well understood, phototherapy seems both to break down bilirubin and to encourage the liver to excrete it from the body. In about 90 to 95 percent of cases of newborn jaundice requiring treatment, phototherapy works to preclude the need for transfusion.

Aside from its dangers, newborn jaundice also holds great fascination as a broad gauge of the child's reaction to environmental stress—whether the stress comes from nature or from humans. Phototherapy itself, for example, came into being when some English nurses observed that those infants in the newborn nursery of their hospital kept closest to the windows and natural light developed less jaundice than children bedded down in the darker reaches of the room. In the United States a few years ago, scattered newborn nurseries experienced severe outbreaks of jaundice when children were exposed to the concentrated fumes of phenol-containing disinfectants after the cleaning staffs of the hospitals switched to these products. There is also some evidence, which has never been thoroughly explored, that the previous use of oral contraceptives may contribute to elevated bilirubin levels.

Jaundice has even provided the final justification for those persons who have all along maintained that the sole thing a newborn wants is to cuddle up with its mother and start nursing—and who were dismissed as sentimentalists for making the claim. It now seems that children fed fairly soon after birth do develop less jaundice than those whose feeding is delayed by a hospital routine that carts them off to nurseries. Moreover, the particular value of jaundice as a gauge of environmental stress is that it broadcasts its presence immediately; it is possible, of course, that some of the agents that provoke jaundice do other harm to the child. The difference is that other damage does not set loose a bile pigment that turns the child yellow—a literal human traffic light signaling "caution."

In no case has this traffic light been more insistent than with jaundice caused by artificial induction; the procedure has now emerged as the single most important "unnatural" cause of jaundice yet identified. But just as it took years for "low-level" lead ingestion to be confirmed as harmful to young minds, so obstetricians were literally performing artificial inductions for decades before the connection with jaundice was perceived. And, just as blood lead levels, the traditional measure of lead absorption, have not essentially defined the risk of brain damage for individual children, so serum bilirubin levels, the traditional measure of degree of jaundice, have also left this individual risk essentially undefined; many children seem unaffected by serum bilirubin levels of 20 mg per 100 ml or more, while some few succumb to severe injury at 6.5 mg.

One of the first really jolting clues to the seriousness of the situation was a 1975 report from St. Mary's Hospital in London. "Jaundice of unexplained aetiology," doctors from St. Mary's complained in *The British Medical Journal*, "is now a serious clinical problem at this hospital, involving not only hazard to infants, but much valuable time of laboratory and medical staff. More infants now require exchange transfusion for unexplained jaundice than for [any other cause.]" As, however, this report proceeded to describe obstetric procedures at St. Mary's, it began to seem that this "unexplained" jaundice epidemic might have a very forthright explanation. In December 1971, St. Mary's had launched what doctors termed a "policy of active management of labor"—meaning that they, rather than the natural course of events, would more and more decide when women delivered their children. Within two years, inductions at St. Mary's had jumped from 15 to 30 percent of births—and with this doubling came another doubling. The percentage of infants with "significant jaundice"—a condition St. Mary's defined as a bilirubin level of 12 mg per 100 ml, or more, in full-term, healthy children—jumped from 8 to 15 percent of live births.

As other hospitals began to similarly compare jaundice among their induced and noninduced babies, their observations paralleled those at St. Mary's. The more people thought about it, the more the association between jaundice and induction seemed not merely logical, but predictable. It has long been known that premature children have both a higher incidence of jaundice than term children and that they succumb to brain injury at generally lower bilirubin levels. Induction, of course, specifically sends children into the world premature to their own inclination to get there; but even inductions done a few days early, with children officially considered full-term, deprive an infant of the full "enzyme surge" that precedes spontaneous labor, including a surge in production of the enzymes involved in bilirubin metabolism.

A few years ago, there was little solid notion of the bilirubin levels threatening to the full-term, healthy child. St. Mary's had defined its worry level as 12 mg; other hospitals might begin worrying at 15 mg and initiate phototherapy at 17 mg; some few institutions were then initiating phototherapy at 10 mg. In 1974, in what appears to be the first follow-up of the later condition of full-term healthy children who, as infants, were jaundiced, the

Swedes reported on some 100 youngsters born between 1957 and 1962; in this relatively small group, they did find a few who had sustained hearing deficits and incoordination from bilirubin levels of about 25 mg. In 1977, working with the huge Perinatal Collaborative population, Dr. Peter Scheidt, a Baltimore pediatrician, documented a trend—although not a statistically significant one—toward delayed motor development in some full-term healthy children whose infant bilirubin levels had been in the range of 10 to 14 mg.

In late 1978, in a move that at least marked an end to "official" approval of elective inductions, the FDA required that the labeling on oxytocin be changed to warn against its use for any but medically needed inductions. Like other such recommendations from the FDA, this one may take years to work its way into medical consciousness; but at least it has been made. The problem of deciding individual danger levels for bilirubin may also be close to being solved. Dr. Audrey Brown, an internationally known authority on infant jaundice associated with Downstate Medical Center in Brooklyn, has, for one, been involved in very promising work with a "hematofluorometer" developed by Bell Laboratories. To put the matter simply, this instrument interprets the extent to which the child's system is "soaked" with bilirubin. (Dr. Brown had also precipiently recommended, as early as 1973, that even full-term healthy children be started on phototherapy when their bilirubin reached 10 mg.)

Although it will never be known for certain how many children were injured by induction, Dr. Peter Dunn, an English pediatrician, who, like other pediatricians, had often found that his work included the care of children left gasping from an induced birth, said in a 1976 *Lancet* article that the belated adverse news about the procedure had not been unexpected. "For some years," he comments, "I have been increasingly dismayed by the amount of birth asphyxia that I suspected but could not prove was iatrogenic [caused by medical procedures or doctors]—and with it there has been a corresponding increase in hypoglycemia and hyperbilirubinemia. Too much bilirubin, too little oxygen, and too little blood glucose: these are the three most important causes of long-term handicap."

✻

According to the Commission on Professional and Hospital Activities, between 1970 and 1976, the American rate of caesarean section, or delivery done by surgical procedure, climbed from 6.1 percent to 11.3 percent of births—and this figure was considered likely to continue climbing at a rate that left even some obstetricians astonished. A professor of obstetrics and gynecology at New York Hospital–Cornell Medical Center has said he expects that, within five years, caesareans could account for one out of three births; the city-wide rate in Akron, Ohio, is already 18 percent of births and, at an obstetric conference a few years ago, one wondering physician noted that the "growing principle seems to be vaginal delivery only of selected patients." He recalled that, at his own hospital in Los Angeles, California, in 1956, when caesareans were still considered an emergency procedure and recognized as by no means minor surgery, the entire obstetrical staff had been placed on probation when the caesarean rate reached 10 percent of births.

The American caesarean rate may have climbed faster than elsewhere, but, in the past decade, most of the industrialized world—except Holland—has experienced a substantial increase in caesarean births. (In Holland, a country that continues to stubbornly resist "modern obstetrics," midwives still deliver all but a few children, anesthesia and other drugs are virtually never employed during vaginal deliveries, the caesarean rate hovers between 2 and 4 percent of births, and about half of births take place at home, rather than in hospitals. Holland has consistently maintained between the second and fourth lowest infant mortality rate on the face of the earth. In the United States, which has medicalized birth as has no other nation, infant mortality not only exceeds that of most of Europe, but also that of Singapore and

Hong Kong. The United States stands eighteenth in world infant mortality.)

With some exceptions, the rise in the rate of caesareans does not seem to be much different from other examples of overmedicalization in the industrialized world; caesareans are a technical feat and many nations now have the equipment, physicians, and affluence on hand to perform unneeded technical feats. Caesareans, however, are a technical feat performed at a junction in life both psychologically and physically delicate for mother and child. They expose the fetus to a range of toxic agents that begins with the plastic that leaches from the bags holding the intravenous solutions administered during all caesareans and ends with powerful anesthetics known full well to cross the placenta and reach the fetal brain. And, according to recent figures from the Los Angeles Women's Hospital, they involve about half of mothers in complications that range from fever to severe bleeding.

For all such reasons, caesareans require strict justification. The traditional justification for a caesarean was simply that the mother's, or more likely the child's, life was in danger. Caesarean rates in the industrialized world have, however, so clearly moved beyond that which is life-saving that any notion current caesarean rates represent a better recognition of true emergencies can be dismissed out of hand. The caesarean situation at St. Mary's—the same London hospital whose jaundice reports were so illuminating—speaks frankly to this point.

In the early 1970s, St. Mary's decided to use internal monitoring on all women who gave birth there—a slightly unusual decision. Most hospitals tend to reserve internal monitoring, which is restrictive and sometimes causes pelvic infections in the mother and scalp infections in the baby, for "high-risk" deliveries. On the other hand, external monitors, which many hospitals prefer for "low-risk" births, seem not to be fully reliable. Like burglar alarms tripped by shadows, they not infrequently send out false indications of fetal distress. In hospital after hospital, the introduction of external monitoring has been associated with marked increases in caesarean deliveries.

In any case, St. Mary's combined internal monitoring with some fairly aggressive other ways of "assessing fetal well-being." In the year from 1973 to 1974, the hospital cut its caesarean rate from 9.6 percent to 5.8 percent of births and, during that same period, slashed its perinatal mortality by 25 percent—from 15.8 to 11.7 per 1000 births. Considering that Dutch midwives seem to be able to keep as good track of fetal well-being with an old-fashioned stethoscope, it seems a shame that St. Mary's had to attach an electrode to the scalp of 92 percent of the children born there to accomplish this. Still, an electrode in the scalp is better than the toxic exposures of an unneeded caesarean, and St. Mary's experience does give some insight into what a "reasonable" caesarean rate might be.

It would actually be reasonable for the United States, which has more precarious teenage pregnancies and other obstetric problems, to have a caesarean rate a few percentage points higher than is common in Western Europe. That the American caesarean rate is so absurdly high, however, would seem to reflect—as does much other overmedicalization in the United States—this nation's uniquely absurd malpractice situation. Parents are now quick to take badly brain-damaged children to court on the claim that the damage was caused by a vaginal delivery. Although it would be exceedingly rare for brain damage to occur during a properly managed vaginal delivery, such claims do have an element of the plausible to them; not all vaginal deliveries, after all, are properly managed. A caesarean delivery, in any case, conclusively eliminates the claim—although it may hardly eliminate brain damage. There is now substantial evidence that the anesthesia exposures during caesareans may leave large numbers of children with delayed motor development and other neurological deficits. The difference is that this evidently more widespread damage is too subtle to become the stuff of court suits; it is virtually impossible to state in an individual case whether a child's slowness in, say, learning to walk is normal to that child or the consequence of anesthetic exposure.

Although conscientious physicians are aware of anesthetic dangers, now that people have won malpractice settlements on the charge, whether valid or not, that their children should have been delivered by caesarean, there is a sense in which all this has moved beyond the restraints good doctors might apply; they are simply losing leeway to balance the occasional freak event against the subtler but evidently more pervasive dangers of anesthesia. "The physician who is more reserved in the approval of fetal monitoring or concerned we are rapidly approaching an era of routine caesarean sections for convenience may be in a legal bind," medical writer Deborah Larned pointed out in the October, 1978, *Ms*. "With strong professional support for monitoring, physicians who do not use the machine may face the possibility of a malpractice suit. Those who use it routinely are in similar jeopardy. Because of the monitors, a tangible record can be offered in court as evidence of 'fetal distress' requiring a caesarean. As Dr. Gerald Stober, a Queens obstetrician, puts it: 'The most common cause of caesareans today is not fetal distress, or maternal distress, but obstetrician distress.' "

It does no good to blame doctors exclusively for this. For whatever reasons, no other country has so basically consented to sacrifice individualized care during birth to the dictates of insurance premiums and malpractice statistics; other countries have panels to weed out frivolous malpractice suits; they don't permit contingency fee systems, which encourage lawyers to pursue cases they perfectly well know to be invalid. They somehow manage without this.

For the society, parents and children alike, the costs of unneeded caesareans appear to be far-ranging. In the first place, caesareans simply cost more money. According to Blue Cross/ Blue Shield, the average bill for a caesarean delivery has now reached about $1,600—double that for a vaginal delivery—and the average eight-day hospital stay for caesareans is, again, double the hospital time associated with vaginal deliveries.

In the second place, caesareans may involve some unique emotional costs. For a good ten years now, there has been substantial animal and human research into the profound, instinctive process of "bonding" between mother and child, which seems to occur in the first few days, but particularly the first hour, after birth. In some species, the mother will never accept or care for a newborn removed from her during that hour. In humans, some observers believe that, during this first hour, undrugged infants and alert mothers follow each other in a "kind of primeval dance," which involves a sequence of mutual gazing and touching motions that seem almost programmed into the subconscious.

The term "primeval dance" comes from Marshall Klaus and John Kennell, who are both professors of pediatrics at the Medical School of Case Western Reserve University. They awakened particular interest in bonding some years ago when they reported the effect of allowing a group of women to keep their babies with them during the first three days of life for several hours longer than the hospital regulations ordinarily permitted. When observed during routine checkups a month later, these women had quite a different way of handling their babies than those whose early contact with their children had been limited to the usual feeding periods. The women with the extra hours were more reluctant to leave their children with someone else and "engaged in significantly more eye-to-eye contact and fondling."

As behavior research in general tends to be, some of the bonding research is quite controversial. Profound love, as witness that between adoptive parents and their children, clearly exists among family members who meet one another somewhat later in life. Nonetheless, no country with the child abuse statistics of the United States is in a position just to throw away any helpful passages nature may have arranged for children and parents to come to terms with one another. Further research has suggested that well-adjusted, middle-class parents tend to overcome a lack of early contact with a child; but for unstable, scared, and poorer parents, careful support and tender care around the time of childbirth—including but not limited to early contact with the baby—can make a tremendous difference in their later attitudes toward the child. Obviously, an unneeded caesarean is not careful, supportive care by any definition. Even though more and more hospitals are enough impressed by the research on bonding that they are trying to get both vaginally and surgically delivered children to their mothers as soon as possible, it is hard to work around the fact that caesareans essentially obliterate early contact. The mothers are anesthetized and being sewn up, and the babies are not infrequently sluggish enough that they are required to spend their first day or two in incubators.

The most important worry that surrounds caesareans, however, is that of toxins—especially anesthesia—reaching the fetus.

The brain at birth is one of the least-finished portions of the body and is destined not only to grow considerably in size during the first few years of life, but to complete much of its structural detail. As far as is known, all agents now commonly used for anesthesia and analgesia (pain relief without rendering someone unconscious) during childbirth cross the placenta and reach the fetal brain—although not always in the same relative concentration or with the same effects. People have, of course, long considered the possibility that anesthesia encounters at birth might interfere with the brain's structural completion; but finding out whether this was so has been a strangely laggard research quest—another example, perhaps, of medicine's reluctance to face potential bad news about its own favored devices.

In 1969, a preliminary analysis of some 400 of the healthiest caesarean children in the Collaborative Perinatal population had shown that about 3 percent more of those exposed to inhalation, rather than "regional," anesthesia at birth were "neurologically abnormal" when they reached their first birthday—the judgment of "neurological abnormality" having been made by giving them a battery of tests. After this solitary, fleeting observation on the possible long-term impact of anesthesia, virtually all work on this question seems to have focused on short-term effects. By the late 1970s, about thirty studies of vaginally delivered children had related various aberrant neurological responses in the first few weeks of life to a variety of obstetrical medications; but no one particularly knew whether such effects eventually faded or not.

The first long-term study to compare various anesthetic and pain-relieving agents in detail is being sponsored by the National Institute of Neurological and Communicative Disorders and Stroke and co-authored by developmental psychologists Yvonne Brackbill and Sarah Broman; it is still underway. In 1979, however, prompted by a Freedom of Information Act suit, the Institute released preliminary information from the huge Brackbill and Broman undertaking. Although some conclusions may be modified as the analysis is completed, the available data do sound a substantial warning against unwarranted drug use during labor and delivery—most especially when the drug in question is inhalation anesthesia. "Despite the increasing number of drugs used during labor and delivery," Brackbill and Broman have written in explanation of their purpose, "there is no empirical evidence bearing on their long-term consequences. The present study seeks to remedy this situation by analyzing the relationship of obstetrical medication to a variety of pediatric/neurological/behavioral measures during the first year of life in a large group of children studied longitudinally."

The population studied, once again, was children in the Collaborative Perinatal Project—specifically the 3500 healthiest children in the project born after uneventful pregnancies and uncomplicated, noninduced deliveries. These children were thought to have been the least likely to have sustained subtle brain damage before birth—whether of genetic or environmental origin—which might confuse or obscure any associations between their drug exposures during childbirth and later neurological deficits. Studies of caesarean children, by contrast, are always open to the chicken-and-egg charge that the children were delivered surgically because there was already something wrong with them. Drs. Brackbill and Broman have, to date, looked at the neurological, behavioral, and physical tests given these children when they were four months, eight months, and one year old; they are proceeding to look at the tests given to the Perinatal Collaborative children at age four.

Even though the children studied were not delivered by

caesarean, there is solid reason to think that Brackbill and Broman's observations about the adverse impact of some agents during vaginal birth also apply during caesarean birth. Two types of agents predominate for both types of deliveries: inhalation anesthesia and the so-called "regional" agents, which are used, in various ways, to block off feeling below the waist while leaving the mother awake. The difference is that generally—although not always—the fetus is exposed to the anesthetic for a shorter time period during a caesarean delivery. (The full caesarean operation takes about three quarters of an hour, but doctors usually remove the baby within eight to ten minutes of the mother's being anesthetized; by contrast, the mean exposure time to inhalation anesthesia among the vaginal mothers Brackbill and Broman studied was 17 minutes.)

With regional anesthesia, Drs. Brackbill and Broman found that lesser doses and shorter exposure times did generally mean that the child later showed fewer neurological aberrations. One of their single most important findings, however, was that with inhalation anesthesia, "neither the dosage, time, nor level was related to outcome." In other words, the inhalation agents caused delayed motor development and other effects even after the briefest of exposures—a finding that makes it doubtful that the relatively shorter fetal contact with these agents during caesarean births lessens their impact on the brain.

Given the particular toxicity of inhalation anesthesia, it is all the more startling that American obstetricians are not just on a binge of performing caesarean deliveries, they are also on a binge of performing them with inhalation agents. In 1970, 32 percent of caesareans carried out in American hospitals involved inhalation anesthesia; by 1975, a survey of teaching hospitals yielded a figure of 43 percent. Since the rate of use of inhalation anesthesia at private hospitals has traditionally been higher than at teaching hospitals, presumably well over half of American caesareans are now being performed with inhalation rather than regional agents.

What may all this specifically mean to the fetus? Some two hundred of the vaginally delivered children Brackbill and Broman studied had been exposed to nitrous oxide—the inhalation agent used during virtually all caesarean deliveries in the United States. Nitrous oxide had the greatest impact on the fetus of any obstetric drug or anesthetic studied—including other inhalation anesthetics, regional agents, and seven "preanesthetic agents," among them narcotics, sedatives, and tranquilizers, also analyzed. The chief impact of nitrous oxide seems to have been in delayed development of the gross motor skills—predominantly attempts to sit, stand, and to move around. Exposure to inhalation anesthesia also seems to have somewhat impaired the concentration and patience of some children; the more difficult the test tasks, the greater the frustration and difficulty some of these children had in trying to cope with them. The inhalation children also tended to be more irritable than children exposed to regionals. (Because so few women in the Collaborative Perinatal Project escaped all exposure to anesthesia, the further comparison of regional children to nonexposed children was not possible.) It was possible, however, to compare the children's relative scores among themselves at ages four months, eight months, and one year. The "neurological abnormalities" of the regional children seemed to be generally fading over time; with the inhalation children, there was no relative improvement in their performance over these months— certainly a strong sign that deficits to them may be permanent.

Certain other findings Brackbill and Broman cite suggest long-term physical effects. At age four months, significantly more children exposed to inhalation anesthesia had fast heart rates and high blood pressure than children exposed to regionals. At this age, 17 percent of inhalation children and 8 percent of regional children had enlarged livers. By age one, although there had been some improvement, more inhalation than regional children still had enlarged livers.

In short, it may be that fetal exposure to inhalation anesthesia considerably strains the body's detoxification system. Concern has also risen about the impact of anesthesia on the immature immunological system. With several—but not all—recent studies showing that children operated on before they are two are later predisposed to allergic disease, particularly in the form of asthma, some observers have begun to wonder whether the early anesthesia exposures attendant to surgery may interfere with "crucial details" of immunologic development. Studies of caesarean children might be a great help in mediating the conflicting opinions about this question. Presumably their very early—actually fetal—exposure to the anesthesia would magnify any later tendency toward allergic diseases.

Now, obviously there are millions of people alive in the world today whose own delivery included an exposure to inhalation anesthesia and who seem indistinguishable from other persons; they hold jobs, love their families, and mow their lawns in season. The question is not essentially one of drastic injury; it is more a question of people's leaving behind little bits of themselves—some part of their patience, their concentration, their coordination, perhaps. The Brackbill and Broman observations should not make women feel irretrievably guilty for asking for pain relief during an excruciating labor. To the extent, however, that most anesthesia and drug use during labor is unnecessary, the Brackbill and Broman observations are a serious indictment. While acknowledging that women in poor nations still customarily give birth without the assistance of drugs, obstetricians often counter that women in the Western world have lost the capacity to put up with pain. But Dutch women are Western women, and 90 percent of them give birth without using drugs.

"In summary," Brackbill and Broman conclude their preliminary observations, "of the more than 3.5 million children born each year in the United States, an increasing number receive anesthetic and pre-anesthetic medications, albeit indirectly [through their mothers]. In addition, each year general anesthetic is administered directly to some 164,000 infants under one year of age and 725,000 children under five years of age. Finally it should be noted that research is now being done on primate fetal surgery, carried out under anesthesia, with the goal of human application.

"Drug administration during the period of brain growth spurt is increasing, and so, presumably, are the attendant problems."

*

All this, of course, is not to say that women don't sometimes need anesthesia during labor; it is not even to say people shouldn't be forgiving of occasional obstetric miscalculations. Because of the unique situation of birth involving two patients at once, when things do go wrong, or look as though they might go wrong, there is often not even the leeway for a few minutes' discussion or thought that exists during other medical procedures. The matter of two patients "puts you in an alarming position," comments Dr. Hilda Pedersen, a specialist in obstetric anesthesia at Columbia-Presbyterian Medical Center. "You have to make decisions in a great hurry which other people can criticize at leisure." An occasional unnecessary caesarean, an occasional induction done in haste for "inadequate" reasons, would seem to be the inevitable accompaniments of the special considerations of birth.

What is not inevitable is that American medicine should be systematically organized to drug and anesthetize the majority of women who give birth when substantial evidence points toward safety lying in just the opposite direction—in systematically encouraging drug-free births whenever feasible.

Is there any way to change the systematic bias toward drugs?

Some people have thought to do it perhaps by "changing" women themselves before they give birth. This approach to more natural labor basically involves training women in the techniques of Lamaze, or "natural" or prepared childbirth. They are taught to control their contractions through breathing exercises and to psychologically control—"psychoprophylaxis" is the formal term—the fear, and even hysteria, that seem as contributory to garbled labors as anything else.

About fifteen years ago, as these techniques began to seriously wend their way to the United States from Europe, the scattered American obstetricians willing to employ them began to report in the medical journals that, aside from the psychological benefits of Lamaze training, it seemed to bolster the physical condition of both mothers and babies; mothers had fewer lacerations and infections and the babies were less likely to be distressed or born prematurely. In June 1978, a group of obstetricians at Northwestern University and Evanston Hospital in Evanston, Illinois, crowned such complimentary observations with their stunning comparison of labor outcome among 500 Lamaze-prepared women and 500 control women matched by age, sex, race, number of children, and educational level. "The LP patients had only one-fourth the number of caesarean sections and one-fifth the incidence of fetal distress," they commented in *Obstetrics and Gynecology*. "Perinatal mortality was one-fourth that of controls, and postpartum infection, measured by both maternal febrile morbidity and the incidence of antibiotic use, was one-third that of controls. . . . Control patients had almost three times as many cases of toxemia of pregnancy—a finding as inexplicable as it is significant—and twice as much prematurity as LP patients."

Although it was not the case in Illinois that Lamaze women received pain relief less frequently than controls—they did, however, receive smaller doses—work elsewhere has further suggested that Lamaze training substantially decreases the need for drugs during labor. The training itself would seem to provide the base; whether this base is used to a large extent seems to depend on whether the attending staff really encourages the women to do without drugs. In a 1975 survey of teaching hospitals, 10 percent of the women giving birth were Lamaze-prepared and 40 percent of them required no drugs during labor.

The better physical condition of mothers and babies, the lower rates of distress, prematurity, and even mortality—and a basis for attempting drug-free births—are no small benefits. Strange to say, however, obstetricians have not generally been enthusiastic about Lamaze training. As of 1976, fewer than 10 percent of pregnant American women had attended certified classes in prepared childbirth and even those numbers had been gained at enormous effort. "The outstanding aspect that has been perennially glossed over," Dr. Clement Yahia, a Massachusetts obstetrician, wrote the *Lancet* a few years ago after it had published an earlier study documenting the physical benefits of Lamaze labors, "is the fact that Lamaze has established a strong foothold in obstetrics in spite of the initial, and for a while, unrestrained, unrelenting and implacable hostility of organized health professionals. . . . The point of this letter is for proper recognition of the pioneering roles that dedicated patients, husbands, nurses, and paramedical personnel played in the face of professional indifference and obstruction. It is quite fashionable these days to say one is having a Lamaze childbirth. A few short years ago Lamaze was a dirty word."

Prepared childbirth is still largely the preserve of articulate and determined women and there is no reason to think that obstetricians generally will push to extend it to others. The present attitude in obstetrics seems to be that Lamaze is fine for middle-class women, or above, but not for poor women, unwed mothers, teenagers, and others judged to be "less than perfect." When asked, for example, to comment on the Evanston findings, Dr. Harold Kaminetzky, who is chairman of Obstetrics and Gynecology at the New Jersey School of Medicine in Newark, told *Medical World News* that Lamaze "might not work so well in places like Harlem Hospital and Martland [Newark City] Hospital, for example, or among unwed mothers and teenagers." Neither Dr. Kaminetzky, nor anyone else, of course, has documented proof that being unwed, or being a teenager or having a baby at Harlem Hospital, automatically renders women incapable of learning breathing exercises. The peculiar tragedy to this thinking is that Lamaze is largely being withheld from the very people who perhaps stand to benefit the most from it; teenage pregnancies are rife with prematurity and trouble and, in the United States, mortality among infants "other than white"—in the language of the Bureau of Vital Statistics—has traditionally been about double that of white children. How can medicine decline to seriously attempt extending to them a technique that—unlike monitoring and unlike drugs—presents no possibility of bad side effects, but does hold the promise of reducing prematurity rates by as much as 50 percent and perinatal mortality by one fourth?

✻

In view of the internal reluctance of obstetrics to change its ways, other people have looked to reform birth practices by actually changing the medical personnel. Dr. Dunn, for one, concluded his *Lancet* article on birth practices and iatrogenic injury to the fetus by advocating that physicians regain "confidence in the normality of the great majority of women and leave them in the care of midwives and husbands." (The presence of a husband, or, presumably, another "support person," during labor seems to as much as halve the need for painkillers.)

By "midwife," Dr. Dunn is not referring to the grandmotherly person of antique image; he is referring to nurses with special training in midwifery. In contradiction, however, to the physician's training, with its emphasis on the perils and dangers of birth, midwifery emphasizes that birth is a natural process that will rarely go wrong when competently aided to follow its own rhythms; midwives are taught to avoid drugs. Surprisingly, in view of the traditional American suspicion of midwifery, a recent major study on fetal well-being done for the National Institutes of Health also recommends that obstetricians turn over low-risk mothers to "a well-trained nurse-midwife." According to the study group, this action would free ample time for doctors, themselves, to deal with pregnant patients who had real problems, while the low-risk patients in the care of "a competent, sympathetic nurse-midwife could get the individual time and attention so necessary to make her pregnancy complete both from an emotional and physical standpoint and not be subject to the harried consultation so characteristic of today's busy obstetrician."✻

✻ No country, including the United States, has enough obstetricians to deliver all its children. Virtually all other nations, except the United States, rich and poor alike, have long tried to fill this gap by training midwives. In the United States, only in about the past five years has there been a concerted effort to train midwives. Large numbers of babies meanwhile have been delivered by a haphazard collection of residents, nurses, and other personnel without much training in obstetrics, a situation that, without doubt, has contributed to infant mortality.

It is here, of course, that the experience of Holland is so instructive. Dutch midwives are not even "well-trained nurse-midwives"; they are further weaned from the temptation to intervene medically in the birth process by a three-year training period that instructs in midwifery alone. Delivering about 90 percent of Dutch babies and rigorously avoiding anesthetics and drugs, they are the mainstay of a very low infant mortality rate.

American doctors bitterly complain of the injustice of comparing infant mortality in the United States, with its teenage mothers, drug addicts, and other obstetric misfits, to that of West European countries. In that case, why not just compare American statistics with those Third World places whose infant mortality is similar to our own? Hong Kong and Singapore now have infant mortality rates slightly below that of the United States; one observes that both localities are crowded, urban places with many poor women and teenage pregnancies. In neither place do doctors deliver a large portion of babies; midwives deliver them—and often with less training than is common for Western midwives.

Hong Kong and Singapore have attained their present infant mortality rates without fetal monitors, caesareans, and the use of fifteen or more separate drugs per pregnancy. Most important, Hong Kong and Singapore are bringing children into the world who are healthy enough to survive on their own; by contrast, the United States has only managed to achieve its present lagging infant mortality rate by making an enormous investment in sophisticated incubators and intensive-care units to keep alive children who are too sickly or premature to immediately survive on their own. Cedars–Sinai Medical Center in Los Angeles, in not untypical figures, reported a few years ago that the in-hospital cost (not counting doctors' fees) of caring for seventy-five infants who had weighed 1000 grams or less at birth was $14,236 apiece for the forty-five who died, and $40,287 apiece for the thirty who survived. Putting things somewhat differently, the hospital noted that about 70 percent of those who survived did appear to be neurologically and developmentally normal at age one to three years. On that basis, "the average adjusted total cost per 'normal' survivor was $88,058."

Hong Kong and Singapore are clearly not places with $88,058 to invest in one normal survivor. Maybe we should study what it is that they are doing to deliver surviving children; maybe we should study the natives and their midwives—or perhaps even take a look at a few of the more wretched corners of our own nation.

Because of the medical hostility to them, the relatively few practicing nurse-midwives in the United States have traditionally concentrated on bringing their services to the leftover women not served by obstetricians—the poorer, out-of-the-way populations who tend to have both higher maternal and infant mortality rates. Their success with these very difficult populations is as much testimony as they need to their reliability and skill. The most comprehensive figures in American nurse-midwifery come from the Frontier Nursing Service, which was founded in 1925 in Leslie County, Kentucky. During the first twenty-five years that they were working in the hard, back hills of Kentucky, the FNS midwives delivered 60 percent of their clients at home—often in cabins lacking both electricity and plumbing. Now most deliveries take place at the Frontier Nursing Service Hospital. (This is not necessarily by choice. Both private and government insurance plans usually decline to pay for home deliveries.) In hospitals or in unheated cabins, however, the FNS has throughout its history maintained a lower rate of "premature births, stillbirths, and neonatal deaths . . . than the national averages." It has also done well by mothers. During its first twenty-five years, its maternal death rate was two thirds lower than the national average for white women, and the service has not lost a single mother in childbirth since 1952.

The Clinica Familiar (Family Clinic) is another outpost of midwifery, again serving women whom conventional obstetrics would brand as "high-risk" mothers. Founded in 1972 by nurse-midwives who are also nuns, the Clinica serves a largely Spanish-speaking population spread over the dusty reaches of Willacy County, Texas, to the edges of the King Ranch. With only one doctor in the county and the nearest hospital with its complex life-support systems an hour away, the midwives at the Clinica Familiar haven't much room for error; they don't seem worried. Prematurity, of course, is often the harbinger not just of infant death but of life-crippling complications. As of 1978, the prematurity rate among deliveries at the Clinica was 4.2 percent, well under the Texas average of 9.3 percent. The average caesarean rate during the first six years of operation was 4.3 percent of deliveries. The Clinica has no fetal monitoring machines.

It is hard not to suspect that the success of midwives is as much psychological as strictly medical. There would appear to be few times in life when self-confidence, an attitude midwives make a great effort to instill, has more bearing on physical health than during pregnancy and childbirth. Sister Angela Murdaugh of the Clinica Familiar has her own view. "We don't call the people who come here 'patients,' " she explains. "We just call them 'the ladies' or 'the mothers.' If you call them patients it sounds as though they're sick. But of course pregnancy is not a sickness. It's an absolutely natural condition."

At the Childbearing Center, a demonstration birth center in Manhattan started a few years ago by the Maternity Center Association, both doctors and midwives partake in the prenatal case of mothers and a pediatrician examines the newborn babies. Women give birth in pleasant rooms, decorated like normal bedrooms, while lying on normal comfortable beds, rather than the cold steel tables of hospital delivery rooms. All clients are required to take prepared childbirth classes and are studiously encouraged to do without drugs. Fewer than 5 percent of the first fifty mothers asked for pain relief during labor. The cost of birth at such centers is about one half to two thirds that of a hospital birth.

The obstetrical establishment has vigorously denounced the Childbearing Center and similar places. When the center was trying to open, the heads of the obstetrical-gynecology departments of every medical school in New York City except Cornell unsuccessfully petitioned the State Department of Health to deny it a license. Still, one suspects that many obstetricians would welcome an alternative to the current situation. In the past, individual doctors could resist fads such as DES and elective induced birth; at present, far from just more and more cutting off the choices of doctors who want to resist caesareans or who would decline to screw an electrode into the scalp of every unborn child, the malpractice explosion is interfering with the ability of doctors to see to the comfort of their patients down to most absurd details. The control that fear of malpractice now has over hospital procedures came as an unpleasant jolt to a woman who recently gave birth at the most expensive hospital in New York City. She went home with a red-haired baby boy, and, actually, quite satisfied with the hospital's service—except for her distinctly black and blue elbows. The reason for them was that during labor she had been stationed in the standard metal hospital bed—the ones with high sides that are reminiscent of cribs for adults. Her elbows kept hitting against the metal sides when she pressed her hands down on her body during contractions; but neither the doctor nor nurse could let down the sides. There was a rule against it. On the million-to-one chance that she might fall out of the bed, the hospital could be sued for malpractice.

For doctors as well as women, birth centers may represent one of the best outs from the increasingly vulturish spectacle of a greedy legal system and a wary hospital establishment trying to outwit one another over the bodies of unborn babies. The choice of a birth center can be protected by women's giving "informed consent" to take the slight risk—if, indeed, it is a risk at all for the normal, healthy mother—of doing without automatic anesthesia, monitoring machines, and unyielding metal beds.

But, of course, to watch what we all accept is as distressing as to watch the current direction of obstetrics. People in the Western world today not only live in more material and physical comfort than their teeming cohabitants on the rest of the planet can even imagine, they also live in more comfort than even the wealthiest and most powerful personages could historically command. A Sun King, in his day, could not purchase polio vaccine any more than a Ming Emperor, in his own time, could have indoor plumbing. All ways of living involve some risks—and it is hardly unfair that they do. But, under these circumstances, to repetitiously risk so much for so little—to risk children and risk the future—seems an act of almost cosmic ingratitude. We would hardly be in a position to call the gods unjust if they took us at our word when we say we are willing to risk genital cancers for the motive of swelling cattle by a few pounds of fat and water, to risk mutations by exposing future genes to X rays that produce no useful diagnostic information, and to risk the neurological development of children for unneeded anesthesia.

*What risks, then, are avoidable and what risks have to be assumed?* Energy, for example, is something people truly need, and all present forms of energy involve some fairly serious health hazards—the paradox being that nuclear energy, which is less hazardous on a day-to-day basis than coal and oil, presents the worst potential hazards from accidents. Although new energy forms may improve the situation sooner than is sometimes thought, and however people choose to deal with this paradox, at the moment, energy is a large factor in the necessary risk equation of technology.

By contrast, the general contamination of something as primary as food is anything but required. Some additives, particularly preservatives, balance their risks with major benefits; but dozens of additives do not. Americans have spent billions to clean up the air; they are now allocating billions more to clean the waterways and yet, as Dr. Epstein points out in *The Politics of Cancer*. food continues to be "the single most important source of exposure to a wide variety of synthetic chemicals, either as direct additives or as accidental contaminants such as pesticides and industrial chemicals."

After serious distinctions between those risks that are necessary and those which are not, the next question is, in blunt terms: *How much real health can you get for a certain amount of money?* James G. Terrill, a Westinghouse analyst, provided a striking example of "cost-benefit" thinking in 1972 when he estimated the relative costs of reducing radiation exposures by equipping all X-ray machines with automatic collimators, or by redesigning nuclear reactors to further contain the relatively small amount of radioactivity they emit (when properly constructed and operated, that is). He was widely accepted as correct when he projected that the use of automatic collimators would cost seven dollars per person (and pennies per X ray as the equipment costs amortize over the years) to guard every individual in the United States from one rem of excess radiation, whereas it would cost between $10,000 and $100,000 per individual to obtain the same radiation reduction by reconstructing nuclear power plants.

It is, perhaps, in balancing benefits against costs that certain medical excesses assume their most bitter edge. If, for instance, it is true that one-third of X-ray exposures are simply part of "defensive medicine," according to a 1975 estimate, Americans that year spent about $1.6 billion to be uselessly exposed to a mutagenic and carcinogenic agent. More grating than the waste represented by these exposures is the vision of the amount of true health a sum like $1.6 billion could purchase. Here is money that would represent an enormous start on cleaning up the Love Canal, and other toxic dumping sites, where the threat of birth defects is very substantial; here is money that could be used to expand the Childhood Lead Control Program from its present concentration in urban areas to towns, such as Chelsea and Somerville, where numerous children fall victim to lead toxicity; here even is money that, in poetic justice, could be used to pay the medical expenses of the some one million children estimated to have been exposed to dangerous head-and-neck X rays.

The amount of money that fetal monitoring concentrates on the last moments of pregnancy similarly seems rather a backward investment, when Americans have yet to properly invest in the early moments of pregnancy. The $25 million that American hospitals spent to purchase fetal monitors in 1976—not to mention the $400 million in extra medical expenses some critics attribute to their use—probably did buy some "statistical health" in the sense of aiding some high-risk babies to be born alive. Money like this, however, could both purchase real health for unborn children and probably keep rather large numbers of them from even becoming high-risk babies. Maternal smoking is the single most important cause of prematurity, along with all its large attendant health risks and huge attendant costs in neonatal care, yet identified. But how many, if any at all, hospitals have smoking-cessation programs for pregnant mothers? Or again, some experts believe that as many as one out of every 500 babies born in the United States suffers some degree of damage from its mother's alcohol consumption. With some of the funds spent on fetal monitoring, hospitals throughout the country could start alcohol treatment programs for pregnant mothers like the one proving so successful at Boston Municipal Hospital. This tactic would not only lead to more children being born live, but to more being born with their brains intact.

Perhaps the final element in retrieving control over environmental hazards involves the fundamental recognition that we are all in this together—a recognition that needs, above all, to find its way into the legal system. As do other questions of social harm, questions of environmental health often find their resolution in the courts. Through the malpractice explosion, the American legal system has lent itself more and more to the notion of simply paying people off for individual bad luck with their health. This same legal system, however, still has great difficulty in contending with the concept of mass threats to health. In various ways, the child and fetus have been strangely caught in these two contradictory trends.

There are few things that will send people to court more

quickly today than the birth of a deformed or brain-injured child. As deserving of sympathy as these children are, the fact remains that there are few things more difficult to prove than where the fault really lies in the case of brain or bodily injury to one youngster. Agents such as thalidomide or DES, which leave behind characteristic patterns of injury, are the exception; for most other suspected teratogens, it is a matter of statistical chance of their involvement in deformities that also occur spontaneously with some frequency. But in this kind of suing, people do not confine themselves to probabilities or even likelihoods. The parents may become almost obsessed with obtaining retribution for what they regard as avoidable injury to their child. The lawyers may proceed on the slimmest of reeds and on the off chance that a defendant will settle out of court in order to avoid the full costs and turmoil of a trial.

To the extent that this is so, the medical backlash in the form of "defensive" medical techniques has in itself become almost an environmental hazard for unborn children. It is not only a major force behind the rising caesarean rate and consequential fetal exposures to anesthesia, it is also pushing to make amniocentesis a commonplace procedure before its safety has been evaluated, and it is propelling all pregnancies toward fetal monitoring. There does not, in short, appear to be any aspect of medical care more subtly or overtly dictated by court decisions than care during pregnancy and childbirth now is.

This does not, of course, solve the problem of malpractice; what stops real malpractice is strict licensing procedures. It does not substantially help in seeing that many malformed children are able to obtain the extra care they need; the more substantial way to help these children and their families, as Dr. Robert Brent, the chairman of pediatrics at Jefferson Medical College, has pointed out in *Teratology*, would be for the society to improve its services to them "so that litigation is no longer necessary to compensate and support families whether negligence is or is not a factor." It may, however, entail widespread health consequences yet to show themselves; had current attitudes prevailed in the late 1940s and a woman then gone to court on the claim that she miscarried because her doctor failed to prescribe DES, would this hormone have been prescribed for virtually all pregnant women in the United States?

In any case, it is chilling to contrast the indulgence of malpractice litigation—which involves questions of harm to one person at a time—with the legal system's longstanding disdain of curbing the use of toxins that may potentially harm millions of people. Both DES and 2,4,5-T, for example, were years ago indicted, condemned, and hanged by the animal—and some human—evidence against them. But both nonetheless survived twenty years of legal challenges to their being added to the food supply or sprayed on millions of persons. Indeed, even with the Oregon miscarriage evidence in hand, the Environmental Protection Agency has just barely managed to sustain its partial ban of 2,4,5-T spraying. Dow Chemical almost immediately filed a motion to have the partial ban stayed—a motion that was heard in federal district court in Bay City, Michigan, by district court judge James Harvey.

Judge Harvey was not at all impressed by the animal evidence against 2,4,5-T or the Oregon miscarriages. In his April 1979 ruling on the Dow motion, he unhesitatingly said he wished he could decide in favor of the chemical corporation and the sole reason he had not done so was that the EPA had not strayed from its statutory power in invoking the ban. "The court will frankly concede that it arrives at this decision with great reluctance," he commented, "and would not in its judgment have ordered the emergency suspensions on the basis of the evidence before the EPA. Nevertheless, EPA has been invested by Congress with broad powers in this area, and the court is not empowered to substitute its judgment for that of EPA."

Not all complainants, of course, win the malpractice cases they bring; and not all malpractice cases are without merit. Nonetheless, in its 1978 ruling that doctors may be liable for the lifetime costs of caring for a malformed child born when they failed to advise parents adequately about prenatal diagnosis, the

New York State Court of Appeals has underlined a stark contrast: in theory, individual physicians are now open to more serious penalties for the birth of a single malformed youngster than have ever been imposed on anyone who manufactured or sprayed 2,4,5-T and its dioxin component—a substance that has evidently been causing miscarriages for years, that is perhaps the single most potent birth-defect-causing agent ever tested in the laboratory, that biologists are coming to view as perhaps the most powerful carcinogen known, and that some observers believe to be responsible for malformations among the children of Vietnam veterans.

One last thing that may help is to remember that the problems now confronting the technological world are not startlingly "new." They were inherent to its formation, and attempts to deal with them—whether well or badly—have been more a continuing part of the human experience than we perhaps sometimes appreciate. People have, for example, contended with "economic" arguments against environmental regulation since Dr. J. Lockhardt Gibson, the Australian who first identified lead paint as a main source of childhood poisoning, found himself attacked for throwing painters out of work. "How any man expressing interest in young children can bring himself, as our master painters bring themselves, to oppose the exclusion of lead from painted surfaces within the reach of young children, passes my comprehension," he wrote in 1919 in the *Medical Journal of Australia.*

Dr. Benjamin Rush, the prominent eighteenth-century physician and signer of the Declaration of Independence, contended with the task of balancing fetal health against the need for treatment during pregnancy. A particular concern to Rush was the then-common use of alcohol to combat morning sickness—a remedy for nausea he presciently considered a danger to the fetus. As a substitute, he advised soda biscuits and patience. In turn, Mary Wollstonecraft, the author of *The Vindication of the Rights of Women,* fought to free the birth process from the useless medical interferences of her own day—including the then rigid practices of confining mothers to their beds for weeks and swaddling newborns in tight wrapping. "It is true," she wrote after doing away with such medical advice during the birth of her first child, "at first [the nurse] was convinced I should kill myself and my child; but since we are both alive and so astonishingly well, she begins to think the Bon Dieu takes care of those who take no care of themselves."

The difference, however, is that the environmental exposures that today's children confront are more numerous in concentration and more toxic in character. Dr. Miller perhaps deserves the last word. He has the commanding perspective of someone with a conservative view on details but an open mind toward the long run. He is not really convinced of the individual hazards implied in many contemporary studies. He does not, as mentioned, believe that prenatal radiation causes childhood cancer; and when queried about the reproductive health of women who work in operating rooms, he is not ready to fully blame anesthesia for their rate of miscarriage and malformed children; these women, he points out, also work under a constant stress perhaps not conducive to successful pregnancies. When, however, asked whether to continue total toxic exposures to the young at their current intensity is to court health disaster, Dr. Miller quietly responds with one word:

"Yes."

# GLOSSARY

ABCC: The Atomic Bomb Casualty Commission.

ABORTIFACIENT: An agent that induces abortion.

ADENOCARCINOMA: A malignant tumor originating in glandular epithelium.

ADENOSIS: The abnormal development of gland tissue.

AGENT ORANGE: A very toxic herbicide widely used in Vietnam.

AMES TEST: A "rapid-assay" system, developed by Dr. Bruce Ames, used to test chemicals for their carcinogenicity.

AMNIOCENTESIS: A technique of prenatal diagnosis mainly used to determine whether a fetus has certain genetic disorders.

ANDROGENS: The male sex hormones.

ANOXIA: Severe deficiency in the amount of oxygen reaching the tissues.

BEIR (Biological Effects of Ionizing Radiation) REPORT: A major report on the biological effects of low-level radiation, first issued by the National Academy of Sciences in 1972. The BEIR Report was somewhat updated in 1977; a major revision is now in preparation.

BHT: Butyleted hydroxytoluene, a common food preservative.

BILIRUBIN: The bile pigment that lends jaundice victims their yellowish hue.

BLASTOCYST: The embryo in its very early stages.

CARCINOGENS: Agents that cause cancer.

CHELATING AGENT: A substance that binds to metals.

CHROMOSOMES: The filamentous structures in the nuclei of cells that contain the genes.

CLEAR-CELL ADENOCARCINOMA: A type of cancer that has characteristically appeared in the vagina and cervix of young women whose mothers were given the synthetic hormone DES during pregnancy.

COAL-TAR DYES: The most commonly used synthetic food colors.

COLLABORATIVE PERINATAL PROJECT: A major study of influences on pregnancy and subsequent infant and child health started in 1957 by the National Institute of Neurological Diseases and Blindness.

CONCEPTUS: A product of conception; embryo.

DBCP: A common abbreviation for dibromochloropropane, a widely used pesticide linked to sterility in some male workers.

DES: A common abbreviation for the synthetic hormone diethylstilbestrol, which caused cancer in the daughters of some women given it as a "pregnancy support."

DIELDRIN: A widely used pesticide.

DIOXIN: A common abbreviation for 2,3,7,8-tetrachlorodibenzo-p-dioxin, or TCDD, an extremely toxic contaminant inevitably created during the manufacture of the herbicide 2,4,5-T.

DNA: Abbreviation for deoxyribonucleic acid, the basic substance of the genes.

DOWN'S SYNDROME: A birth defect, also known as *mongolism,* caused by chromosome damage and characterized by subnormal intelligence.

EDTA: A chelating agent used to treat lead-exposed children, which is also employed as a food additive.

EPIDEMIOLOGY: The study of the incidence and causation of disease in populations.

ESTROGENS: Female sex hormones produced by the ovaries.

FDA: The Food and Drug Administration.

FETAL ALCOHOL SYNDROME: Prenatal injury from chronic maternal alcohol consumption characterized by brain damage and craniofacial abnormalities in the fetus. Abbreviated FAS.

FNS: The Frontier Nursing Service.

FRC: The Federal Radiation Council (now defunct).

GAMETES: Mature sex, or germ, cells; the eggs and sperm.

HEMOGLOBIN: The iron-containing protein pigment in the red blood cells that transports oxygen.

HEPTACHLOR: An insecticide.

HEXACHLOROPHENE: An antibacterial agent now limited in distribution because of its toxicity.

HODGKIN'S DISEASE: A malignant disease of the lymph system; about half its victims are under age twenty-five.

HORMONE SUPPORTS: Both natural and synthetic sex hormones, once widely prescribed for pregnant women in the mistaken belief that they could prevent miscarriage and pregnancy complications.

HYPERACTIVE: Pathologically overactive.

HYPERBILIRUBINEMIA: The presence of too much *bilirubin* (q.v.) in the blood.

HYPERKINESIS: Abnormally heightened, purposeless muscular activity; often used interchangeably with *hyperactivity* although not a precise synonym.

HYPOGLYCEMIA: Too little glucose (blood sugar).

IATROGENIC: Caused by physicians or medical procedures.

IONIZING RADIATION: The radiation category that includes gamma rays and X rays; radiation sufficiently strong to dislodge electrons from atoms.

JAUNDICE: A disease symptom characterized by a yellowish cast to the skin and usually a sign of abnormality in the liver, gallbladder, or red blood cells; caused by *hyperbilirubinemia* (q.v.).

LAMAZE TECHNIQUE: A method of natural childbirth almost

universally used in Russia and China and introduced to the West by the late French obstetrician Fernand Lamaze.

LIDOCAINE: A local anesthetic.

LIMB REDUCTION DEFECT: Congenital full or partial loss of the extremities; a birth defect.

LOW-LEVEL RADIATION: A term without precise definition, but often used to refer to radiation doses of less than ten *rads* (see *rad*).

METHYLMERCURY: A mercury compound known for causing *Minamata disease* (q.v.).

MICROGRAM: One millionth of a gram.

MICROPHALLUS: An undersized penis.

MICROWAVES: A type of low-frequency electromagnetic radiation.

MILLILITER: One thousandth of a liter; a metric unit of volume.

MILLIRAD: One thousandth of a *rad* (q.v.).

MINAMATA DISEASE: A degenerative disease first noticed among residents of the village of Minamata, Japan, who had eaten fish contaminated with *methylmercury*.

MONGOLISM: A birth defect now usually known as *Down's syndrome* (q.v.).

NEOPLASIA: Abnormal growths, either benign or malignant.

NEURAL TUBE DEFECTS: A group of central nervous system defects thought to result from abnormal development of the embryonic neural tube.

NIOSH: National Institute of Occupational Safety and Health.

NITROSAMINES: A class of highly carcinogenic compounds that, under some circumstances, may form from nitrites, including nitrite preservatives.

NITROUS OXIDE: An inhalation anesthetic.

NYSTAGMUS: Rapid, involuntary movements of the eyeballs.

OOCYTES: Immature eggs.

ORGANOCHLORINE: Any compound formed of chlorine and organic elements; DDT is an organochlorine pesticide.

ORGANOGENESIS: The main period of embryonic organ development.

PCBs: Abbreviation for polychlorinated biphenyls, a group of widely used industrial chemicals.

PELVIMETRY: An X-ray examination done to determine the relative size of the maternal pelvis and the fetal head. The term can also refer to any measurement of the dimensions of the pelvis.

PLACENTA: The organ uniting the fetus to the maternal uterus.

PLATELETS: Small cellular bodies in the blood that plug internal tears in the capillaries and small blood vessels.

PPB: Parts per billion.

PPM: Parts per million.

PROGESTERONE: A natural progestational hormone.

PROGESTINS: Progestational hormones. Progesterone, the primary natural progestin, and various synthetic progestins were once widely prescribed as *hormone supports* (q.v.) during pregnancy.

PROSTAGLANDINS: Substances synthesized within the cells by the action of certain enzymes; among other things, they help regulate gestation and labor.

PSEUDOHERMAPHRODITISM: Having the reproductive gonads of one sex and the external genitals of the other.

PSYCHOPROPHYLAXIS: Prevention of pain or discomfort by mental attitude and training.

RAD: Abbreviation for "radiation absorbed dose," a measure of X-ray energy absorbed per gram of tissue.

RELATIVE BIOLOGICAL EFFECTIVENESS (RBE): "Quality" factors used to compare the biological effects of absorbed doses of different types of ionizing radiation.

REM: Abbreviation for "roentgen equivalent man," a unit of radiation measure used to compare dose-effects from different types of ionizing radiation.

SENSORIMOTOR DEFICITS: Problems in motor and sensory function.

SPERM COUNT: A measure of the number of sperm cells per milliliter of ejaculate; one indice of fertility.

SPINA BIFIDA: A central nervous system defect in which the spinal column does not fully close and the child may be severely crippled.

SQUAMOCOLUMNAR JUNCTION: The region in the cervix where the columnar epithelium typical of the uterus meets the squamous lining of the vagina.

STILBESTEROL: *DES* (q.v.).

STILLBIRTH: A child born dead.

SUPEROVULATE: To ovulate (or release eggs) excessively.

TERATOGEN: An agent that causes defective form or structure in the fetus.

TRANSPLACENTAL CARCINOGEN: A cancer-causing agent that traverses the placenta to assault the fetus.

2,4,5-T: A herbicide still being used in the United States and once widely used in Vietnam as a component of Agent Orange.

VINYL CHLORIDE: A synthetic material, sometimes plasticized, widely used in consumer and industrial products.

X CHROMOSOME: The larger sex chromosome, found in all female eggs and half of all male sperm cells; a female normally has two X chromosomes.

Y CHROMOSOME: The smaller sex chromosome, which in man confers maleness; a male normally has one X and one Y chromosome.

ZYGOTE: A fertilized egg.

# NOTES

*The following notes, which are arranged according to page by chapter, cite the major studies, research, and articles referred to in the text. Virtually all direct quotes not otherwise identified have come from personal or telephone interviews.*

## CHAPTER ONE

**p. 4** Carson, Rachel, *Silent Spring.* New York: Fawcett Crest Edition, 1967, p. 168.

**p. 5** *Biological Effects of Ionizing Radiation (BEIR Report).* Washington, D.C.: National Academy of Sciences, 1972, p. 63.

**p. 6** Hertig, A., *et al.,* "A Description of 34 Human Ova Within the First 17 Days of Development." *American Journal of Anatomy* 98:435–59, 1956.

Gordon, H. L., "An Industry Viewpoint." *Proceedings of a Conference on Women and the Workplace.* Washington, D.C.: The Society for Occupational and Environmental Health, 1977, p. 120.

"Eight Oregon Women Seek Link of Herbicide to Miscarriages." *Washington Post,* August 15, 1978, p. A3.

**p. 7** Carr, D. H., "Chromosomes and Abortion." *Advances in Human Genetics* 2:201–49, 1971.

Legator, M., and S. Rinkus, "The Chemical Environment and Mutagenesis." *Proceedings of a Conference on Women and the Workplace, op. cit.,* pp. 5–20.

**p. 8** Herbst, A. L., H. Ulfelder, and D. C. Poskanzer, "Adenocarcinoma of the Vagina: Association of Maternal Stilbestrol Therapy with Tumor Appearance in Young Women." *New England Journal of Medicine* 284:878–81, 1971.

Michael, P., *Tumors of Infancy and Childhood.* Philadelphia: J. B. Lippincott, 1964, p. 1

p. 10   Smith, A., "Congenital Minamata Disease." *Proceedings of a Conference on Women and the Workplace, op. cit.,* pp. 75–83.

Spyker, J., "Assessing the Impact of Low-level Chemicals on Development: Behavioral and Latent Effects." *Federation Proceedings* 34:1835–44, 1975.

p. 12   Dunn, H. G., *et al.,* "Maternal Smoking During Pregnancy and the Child's Subsequent Development." *Canadian Journal of Public Health* 68:43–50, 1977.

p. 13   Jones, H. W., and L. Wilkins, "The Genital Anomaly Associated with Prenatal Exposure to Progestogens." *Fertility-Sterility* 11:148–56, 1960.

Bibbo, M., W. B. Gill, F. Azizi, *et al.,* "Follow-up Study of Male and Female Offspring of DES-exposed Mothers." *Journal of Obstetrics and Gynecology* 49:1–8, 1977.

p. 14   Reinisch, J. M., and W. G. Karow, "Prenatal Exposure to Synthetic Progestins and Estrogens." *Archives of Sexual Behavior* 6:257–88, 1977.

p. 15   Hunt, V. R., and W. L. Cross, "Infant Mortality and the Environment of a Lesser Metropolitan County." *Environmental Research* 9:135–51, 1975.

p. 16   Kane, D. N., "The Air Children Breathe." *The Nation,* August 28, 1976, p. 143.

Finberg, L., "Interaction of the Chemical Environment with the Infant and Young Child." *Pediatrics* (Suppl.) 53:831–36, 1974.

p. 18   Brodeur, P., *The Zapping of America.* New York: W. W. Norton and Company, 1977, pp. 81–84.

p. 23   Benirschke, K., *et al.,* "Genetic Diseases." *Prevention of Embryonic, Fetal and Perinatal Disease,* Vol. 3. Washington, D.C.: Fogarty International Center, National Institutes of Health, 1976 (HEW Publication No. NIH 76-853), p. 223.

p. 24   Uchida, I., "Epidemiology of Mongolism: the Manitoba Study." *Annals of the New York Academy of Sciences* 171:361–69, 1970.

Linsjö, A., "Down's Syndrome in Sweden." *Acta Paediatrica Scandinavica* 63:571–76, 1974.

Shiono, H., *et al.,* "Maternal Age and Down's Syndrome." *Clinical Pediatrics* 14:241–44, 1975.

Gardner, R. J., *et al.,* "A Survey of 972 Cytogenetically Examined Cases of Down's Syndrome." *New Zealand Medical Journal* 78:403–9, 1973.

Janerich, D. T., *et al.,* Down's Syndrome and Oral Contraceptive Usage." *British Journal of Obstetrics and Gynecology* 83:617–20, 1976.

p. 25   Colemann, R. D., and A. Stoller, "A Survey of Mongoloid Births in Victoria, Australia." *American Journal of Public Health* 52:813–29, 1962.

Lowry, R. D., *et al.,* "Down's Syndrome in British Columbia, 1952–1973." *Teratology* 14:29–34, 1976.

p. 26   Meselson, M., Foreword: *Chemical Mutagens.* A. Hollaender, ed. New York: Plenum Press, 1971, p. *ix.*

*Medical World News,* April 26, 1968, p. 27.

p. 27   Muller, H. G., "Our Load of Mutations." *American Journal of Human Genetics* 2:111–76, 1950.

Neel, J. V., "The Detection of Increased Mutation Rates in Human Populations." *Mutagenic Effects of Environmental Contaminants,* H. E. Sutton and M. I. Harris, eds. New York: Academic Press, 1972, pp. 99–119.

**p. 28** Neel, J. V., "A Note on Congenital Defects in Two Unacculturated Indian Tribes." *Congenital Defects*, D. Janerich, *et al.*, eds. New York: Academic Press, 1974, pp. 3–15.

Didion, J., *Slouching Towards Bethlehem*. New York: Delta Dell Edition, 1978, p. 146.

*CHAPTER TWO*

**p. 31** Warkany, J., "Trends in Teratologic Research." *Pathobiology of Development*, E. Perrin and M. Finegold, eds. Baltimore: Williams and Wilkins, 1972, pp. 1–10.

**p. 32** Wilson, J. G., *The Environment and Birth Defects*. New York: Academic Press, 1973, pp. 48–50.

**p. 34** Fedrick, J., "Anencephalus and Local Water Supply." *Nature* 227:176–77, 1970.

Roberts, C. J., and R. G. Powell, "Interrelation of the Common Congenital Malformations." *Lancet*. November 1, 1975, pp. 848–50.

Lowe, C., "Congenital Malformations and the Problem of Their Control." *British Medical Journal* 3:515–20, 1972.

**p. 35** Tuchmann-Duplessis, H., "Teratogenic Screening Methods." *Acta Endocrinologica* (Suppl.) 185:203–19, 1974.

**p. 36** Infante, P. F., "Oncogenic and Mutagenic Risks in Communities with Polyvinyl Chloride Production Facilities." *Annals of the New York Academy of Sciences* 271:49–52, 1976.

Infante, P. F., J. K. Wagoner, A. J. McMichael, *et al.*, "Genetic Risks of Vinyl Chloride." *Lancet*, April 3, 1976, pp. 734–39.

Edmonds, L. D., H. Falk, and J. E. Nissim, Letter: "Congenital Malformations and Vinyl Chloride." *Lancet*, November 29, 1975, p. 1098.

**p. 37** "Upstate Waste Site May Endanger Lives." *New York Times*, August 2, 1978, p. A1.

Nailor, M. G., *et al.*, eds., *Love Canal: Public Health Time Bomb*. Albany, New York: New York State Department of Health, September 1978.

**p. 38** Paigen, B., "Health Hazards at Love Canal; Testimony to the House Subcommittee on Oversight and Investigations." March 21, 1979.

**p. 39** Brown, M., "Love Canal, U.S.A." *New York Times Magazine*, January 21, 1979, p. 23.

Jones, N. F., "Residence Under an Airport Landing Pattern as a Factor in Teratism. *Archives of Environmental Health* 33:10–12, 1978.

Zaret, M., Letter: "Teratogenic Airports?" *Medical World News*, June 26, 1978.

**p. 40** Brodeur, P., *The Zapping of America*, New York: W. W. Norton and Company, 1977, pp. 135–46.

**p. 41** Saxen, I., and A. Lahti, "Cleft Lip and Palate in Finland." *Teratology* 9:217–24, 1974.

**p. 42** Warner, R. H., and H. L. Rossett, "The Effects of Drinking on Offspring: An Historical Survey of the British and American Literature." *Journal of Studies on Alcohol* 36:1395–420, 1975.

p. 44 Jones, K., D. Smith, C. Ulleland, et al., "Pattern of Malformation in Offspring of Chronic Alcoholic Mothers." Lancet, June 9, 1973, pp. 1267-71.

Ouellette, E. M., H. L. Rossett, N. P. Rosman, et al., "Adverse Effects on Offspring of Maternal Alcohol Abuse During Pregnancy." New England Journal of Medicine, September 8, 1977, pp. 528-30.

p. 45 "Pregnancy and Booze Don't Mix, Warns U.S." New York Post, February 9, 1979, p. 8.

p. 47 American Society of Anesthesiologists, "Occupational Disease Among Operating Room Personnel: A National Study." Anesthesiology 41:321-40, 1974.

p.48 Knill-Jones, R. P., et al., "Anesthetic Practice and Pregnancy: Controlled Survey of Male Anesthetists in the United Kingdom." Lancet, October 25, 1975, pp. 807-9.

Cohen, E. N., et al., "A Survey of Anesthetic Health Hazards Among Dentists." Journal of the American Dental Association 90:1291-96, 1975.

p. 49 Nora, J. J., and A. H. Nora, Letter: "Birth Defects and Oral Contraceptives." Lancet, April 28, 1973, pp. 941-42.

p.50 Nora, A. H., and J. J. Nora, "A Syndrome of Multiple Congenital Anomalies." Archives of Environmental Health 30:17-21, 1975.

Janerich, D. T., et al., "Oral Contraceptives and Congenital Limb Reduction Defects." New England Journal of Medicine 291:697-700, 1974.

Smith, E. S., et al., "An Epidemiological Study of Congenital Reduction Deformities of the Limbs." British Journal of Preventive and Social Medicine 31:39-41, 1977.

Shapiro, S., "Evidence Concerning Possible Teratogenic Effects of Exogenous Female Hormones; Testimony to the House Select Committee on Population." August 9, 1978.

p. 52 Harlap, S., et al., Letter: "Birth Defects and Estrogens and Progesterones in Pregnancy." Lancet, March 22, 1975, pp. 682-83.

p. 54 Simpson, W. J., "A Preliminary Report on Cigarette Smoking and the Incidence of Prematurity." American Journal of Obstetrics and Gynecology 73:808-15, 1957.

Meyer, M. B., J. A. Tonascia, and C. Buck, "The Interrelationship of Maternal Smoking and Increases in Perinatal Mortality with Other Risk Factors." American Journal of Epidemiology 100:443-51, 1974.

Meyer, M. B., B. S. Jonas, and J. A. Tonascia, "Perinatal Events Associated with Maternal Smoking During Pregnancy." American Journal of Epidemiology 103:464-76, 1976.

Meyer, M. B., and J. A. Tonascia, "Maternal Smoking, Pregnancy Complications and Perinatal Mortality." American Journal of Obstetrics and Gynecology 128:494-502, 1977.

p. 56 Butler, N. R., and H. Goldstein, "Smoking in Pregnancy and Subsequent Child Development." British Medical Journal 2:573-75, 1973.

p. 57 Heinonen, O. P., D. Sloane, and S. Shapiro, eds., Birth Defects and Drugs in Pregnancy. Littleton, Mass.: Publishing Sciences Group, 1977, pp. viii, 264-65.

**p.58**  Warkany, J., "Congenital Malformations Through the Ages." *Drugs and Fetal Development,* M. A. Klingsberg, ed. New York: Plenum, 1972, p. 46.

Bleyer, W. A., and R. T. Breckenridge, "Studies on the Detection of Adverse Drug Reactions in the Newborn." *Journal of the American Medical Association* 213:2049–53, 1970.

**p. 59**  Turner, G., and E. Collins, "Maternal Effects; Fetal Effects of Regular Salicylate Ingestion in Pregnancy." *Lancet,* August 23, 1975, pp. 335–38, 338–39.

Shapiro, S., *et al.,* "Perinatal Mortality and Birth-weight in Relation to Aspirin Taken During Pregnancy." *Lancet,* June 26, 1976, pp. 1375–76.


## CHAPTER THREE

**p. 64**  Jacobson, M. F., *Eater's Digest.* New York: Anchor Books, 1972, p. 35.

Allen, J. R., *et al.,* "Responses of Rats and Nonhuman Primates to 2,5,2′,5′-Tetrachlorobiphenyl." *Environmental Research* 9:265–73, 1975.

McCann, J., and B. N. Ames, "The Detection of Mutagenic Metabolites of Carcinogens in Urine with the *Salmonella*/Microsome Test." *Annals of the New York Academy of Sciences* 269:21–25, 1975.

**p. 65**  Maugh, T. H. II, "Chemical Carcinogens: The Scientific Basis for Regulation." *Science,* September 29, 1978, pp. 1200–5.

**p. 66**  Legator, M. S., and S. J. Rinkus, "The Chemical Environment and Mutagenesis." *Proceedings of a Conference on Women and the Workplace,* Washington, D.C.: The Society for Occupational and Environmental Health, 1977, pp. 5–20.

Shephard, T. H., *A Catalog of Teratogenic Agents.* Baltimore, Md.: Johns Hopkins University Press, 1976.

**p. 68**  "How Smoking or Drugs Damage the Fetus." *Medical World News,* May 31, 1976, p. 50.

**p. 70**  Warburton, D., J. Kline, Z. Stein, *et al.,* Letter: "Trisomy Cluster in New York." *Lancet,* July 23, 1977, p. 201.

**p. 73**  Dr. Miller quoted in Wright, L., "Troubled Waters." *New Times,* May 13, 1977, p. 38.

Stone, D., E. Matalka, and J. Riordan, "Hyperactivity in Rats Bred and Raised on Relatively Low Amounts of Cyclamates." *Nature* 224:1326–8, 1969.

Stone, D., *et al.,* "Can Artificial Sweeteners Ingested in Pregnancy Affect the Offspring?" *Nature* 231:53, 1971.

**p. 74**  Corbett, T., "Cancer, Miscarriages and Birth Defects Associated with Operating Room Exposure." *Proceedings of a Conference on Women and the Workplace, op. cit.,* pp. 94–99.

**p. 75**  Ferstandig, L. J., "Trace Concentrations of Anesthetic Gases: A Critical Review of Their Disease Potential." *Anesthesia and Analgesia* 57:328–45, 1978.

"Birth Defects and Their Environmental Causes." *Medical World News,* January 22, 1971, pp. 54–55.

**p. 78**  Carr, D. H., "Chromosome Studies in Selected Spontaneous Abortions:

Conception After Oral Contraceptives." *Canadian Medical Association Journal* 103:343–50, 1970.

Janerich, D. T., J. M. Piper, D. M. Glebatis, "Oral Contraceptives and Congenital Limb Reduction Defects." *New England Journal of Medicine* 291:697–700, 1974.

**p. 79** Petrovski quoted in Seaman, B., and G. Seaman, *Women and the Crisis in Sex Hormones*. New York: Rawson Associates, 1977, p. 61.

Harlap, S., In press.

Harlap, S., and A. M. Davies, *The Pill and Births: The Jerusalem Study* (Part I: Text). Jerusalem, 1978, p. 6.

Rothman, K. J., and C. Lonik, "Oral Contraceptives and Birth Defects." *New England Journal of Medicine* 299:522–23, 1978.

**p. 80** Bross, I. J., Letter: "Oral Contraceptives and Birth Defects." *New England Journal of Medicine* 300:47, 1978.

Harlap and Davies, *The Pill and Births: The Jerusalem Study* (Part I: Text), *op. cit.,* p. 119.

**p. 84** "An Assessment of the Hazards of Amniocentesis: Report of the M.R.C. Working Party on Amniocentesis." *British Journal of Obstetrics and Gynecology,* Vol. 85 (Suppl. 2), 1978.

Golbus, M. S., W. D. Loughman, C. J. Epstein, *et al.,* "Prenatal Genetic Diagnosis." *New England Journal of Medicine* 162:157–63, 1979.

**p. 85** Scheidt, P. C., and F. E. Lundin, "Investigations for Effects of Intrauterine Ultrasound in Humans." *Symposium on Biological Effects and Characterizations of Ultrasound,* Rockville, Md.: Bureau of Radiological Health, 1977 (HEW Publication FDA-78-8048), pp. 19–26.

Scheidt, P. C., F. Stanley, and D. A. Bryla, "One-year Follow-up of Infants Exposed to Ultrasound in Utero." *American Journal of Obstetrics and Gynecology* 131:743–48, 1978.

**p. 86** Editorial: "The Risk of Amniocentesis." *Lancet,* December 16, 1978, pp. 1287–88.

## CHAPTER FOUR

**p. 90** "Readin', Writin' (and Druggin')." *New York Times,* October 19, 1975, p. IV-13.

Lockey, S. D., "Reactions to Hidden Agents in Foods, Beverages and Drugs." *Annals of Allergy* 29:461–66, 1971.

Randolph, T. G., "Allergy as a Causative Factor of Fatigue, Irritability, and Behavior Problems of Children." *Journal of Pediatrics* 31:560–72, 1947.

**p. 93** Williams, J. I., D. M. Cram, F. T. Tansig, *et al,* "Relative Effects of Drugs and Diet on Hyperactive Behaviors." *Pediatrics* 61:811–17, 1978.

Harley, J. P., R. S. Ray, L. Tomasi, *et al,* "Hyperkinesis and Food Additives: Testing the Feingold Thesis." *Pediatrics* 61:818–28, 1978.

Bierman, C. W., and C. T. Furukawa, Commentary: "Food Additives and Hyperkinesis: Are There Nuts Among the Berries?" *Pediatrics* 61:932–33, 1978.

**p. 95** David Hathaway quoted in *Washington Star,* September 12, 1975, p. A1.

Letter to Dr. B. Feingold from G. B. Gladman, Administrator, Brant Sanitorium, October 1, 1975.

**p. 97** Jacobson, M. F., *Eater's Digest.* New York: Anchor Books, 1972, p. 56.

Jenkins, J., and J. Jenkins, "The Chemical Fast." *Environmental Action,* November 19, 1977, pp. 4–7.

Conners, C. K., C. H. Goyette, D. A. Southwick, *et al.,* "Food Additives and Hyperkinesis." *Pediatrics* 58:154–66, 1976.

**p. 100** Shaywitz, B. A., *et al.,* Abstract: "The Effects of Chronic Administration of Food Colorings on Activity Levels and Cognitive Performance in Normal and Hyperactive Developing Rat Pups." *Annals of Neurology* 4:196, 1978.

Gellis, S. S., *Pediatric Notes,* September 11, 1978.

**p. 101** Pihl, R. O., and M. Parkes, "Hair Element Content in Learning Disabled Children." *Science,* October 14, 1977, pp. 204–6.

**p. 102** Ott, J. N., "The Eyes' Dual Function" (Part 2). *Eye, Ear, Nose and Throat* 53:24–35, 1974.

**p. 104** Berry, J. W., *Chemical Villains.* St. Louis: 1974, p. 75.

**p. 106** Lin-Fu, J. S., "Vulnerability of Children to Lead Exposure and Toxicity." *New England Journal of Medicine* 289:1229–33, 1289–93, 1973.

**p. 108** de la Burdé, B., and M. S. Choate, Jr., "Does Asymptomatic Lead Exposure in Children have Latent Sequelae?" *Journal of Pediatrics* 81:1088–91, 1972.

de la Burdé, B., and M. S. Choate, Jr., "Early Asymptomatic Lead Exposures and Development at School Age." *Journal of Pediatrics* 87:638–42, 1975.

**p. 110** Chisolm, J. J., Jr., "Is Lead Poisoning Still a Problem?" *Clinical Chemistry* 23:252–55, 1977.

**p. 111** Beattie, A. D., *et al.,* "Role of Chronic Low-level Lead Exposure in the Aetiology of Mental Retardation." *Lancet,* March 15, 1975, pp. 589–92.

**p. 112** David, O. J., S. P. Hoffman, J. Sverd, *et al.,* "Lead and Hyperactivity: Behavioral Response to Chelation." *American Journal of Psychiatry* 133:1155–58, 1976.

David, O. J., S. P. Hoffman, B. McGann, *et al.,* "Low Lead Levels and Mental Retardation." *Lancet,* December 25, 1976, pp. 1376–79.

**p. 113** David, O. J., Letter: "The Food Additive Hypothesis, Lead and Hyperactivity." *Pediatrics* 57:576, 1976.

Needleman, H. L., C. Gunnoe, A. Leviton, *et al.,* "Deficits in Psychological and Classroom Performance of Children with Elevated Dentine Lead Levels." *New England Journal of Medicine* 300:689–95, 1979.

**p. 116** Summarized in Lerner, M., and C. Johnston, *Tomorrow's Children,* Bolinas, Cal.: Commonweal, 1976, pp. 106–8.

**p. 119** Newell, G. R., *et al.,* "Case-control Study of Hodgkin's Disease." *Journal of the National Cancer Institute* 51:1437–41, 1973.

**p. 121** Letter to Dr. Benjamin Feingold from Dr. H. Jerome Crampton, August 4, 1977.

## CHAPTER FIVE

p. 125 Anderson, H. A., R. Lilis, S. M. Daum, et al., "Household Contact Asbestos and Neoplastic Risk." *Annals of the New York Academy of Sciences* 271:311-23, 1976.

p. 127 Smith, O. W., and G. Smith, "The Influence of Diethylstilbestrol on the Progress and Outcome of Pregnancy." *American Journal of Obstetrics and Gynecology* 58:994-1009, 1949.

Smith, O. W., "Diethylstilbestrol in the Prevention and Treatment of Pregnancy Complications." *American Journal of Obstetrics and Gynecology* 56:821-34, 1948.

p. 128 Herbst, A. L., H. Ulfelder, and D. C. Poskanzer, "Adenocarcinoma of the Vagina." *New England Journal of Medicine* 284:878-81, 1971.

p. 130 Stafl, A., "Clinical Detection of Vaginal Adenosis and Clear-cell Adenocarcinoma." *Journal of Reproductive Medicine* 15:19-24, 1975.

"DES Daughters: No Rise in Squamous Dysplasia or Cancer." *Medical World News,* April 17, 1978, pp. 7-8.

Herbst, A. L., P. Cole, T. Colton, et al., "Age-incidence and Risk of Diethylstilbestrol-related Clear-cell Adenocarcinoma of the Vagina and Cervix." *American Journal of Obstetrics and Gynecology* 128:43-50, 1977.

p. 131 Dieckmann, W. J., et al., "Does the Administration of Diethylstilbestrol During Pregnancy Have Therapeutic Value?" *American Journal of Obstetrics and Gynecology* 66:1062-81, 1953.

p. 132 Wolfe, S., Letter to HEW Secretary Joseph Califano, December 12, 1977. (Health Research Group, Washington, D.C.)

Bibbo, M., W. M. Haenszel, G. L. Wied, et al., "A Twenty-five Year Follow-up Study of Women Exposed to Diethylstilbestrol During Pregnancy." *New England Journal of Medicine* 298:763-67, 1978.

p. 133 Bibbo, M., W. B. Gill, F. Azizi, et al., "Follow-up Study of Male and Female Offspring of DES-exposed Mothers." *Journal of Obstetrics and Gynecology* 49:1-8, 1977.

p. 135 Schottenfeld, D., Memorial Sloan-Kettering Cancer Center: Unpublished data.

"DES Task Force Summary Report." Washington, D.C.: Office of the Secretary of HEW, 1978.

p. 138 "Diethylstilbestrol." *Medical World News,* August 23, 1976, pp. 44-56.

Fishbane, F., Lecture: "Emotional Problems in the DES Exposed." 1978.

p. 142 Wolfe, S., Statement to FDA Ob-Gyn Advisory Committee, January 30, 1978. Washington, D.C.: Health Research Group Publication 516, 1978.

p. 144 Wolfe, S., Letter to HEW Secretary F. David Mathews, December 9, 1975. Washington, D.C.: Health Research Group Publication 353.

p. 145 Ulfelder, H., "Stilbestrol, Adenosis, and Adenocarcinoma." *American Journal of Obstetrics and Gynecology* 117:794-800, 1973.

p. 147 Napalkov, N. P., "The Problem of Transplacental Carcinogenesis." *Transplacental Carcinogenesis,* L. Tomatis and U. Mohr, eds. Lyons: IARC Scientific Publication No. 4, 1973, pp. 1-13.

**p. 147** Tanaka, T., "Transplacental Induction of Tumors and Malformations in Rats Treated with Some Chemical Carcinogens." *Transplacental Carcinogenesis,* pp. 100–11.

**p. 148** Rice, J., "An Overview of Transplacental Carcinogenesis." *Teratology* 8:113–26, 1973.

Gardner, H., "Sowbelly Blues." *Esquire,* November 1977, p. 112.

**p. 150** Spark, R. F., "Legislating Against Cancer." *New Republic,* June 3, 1978, p. 16.

"Study on Saccharin Said to Seek Curbs." *New York Times,* February 28, 1979, p. A1.

**p. 152** Pitkin, R. M., *et al.,* "Placental Transmission and Fetal Distribution of Saccharin." *American Journal of Obstetrics and Gynecology* 111:280–86, 1971.

**p. 153** Epstein, S., *The Politics of Cancer.* San Francisco: Sierra Club Books, 1978, p. 195.

Ineke, C., P. Neutel, and C. Buck, "Effect of Smoking During Pregnancy on the Risk of Cancer in Children." *Journal of the National Cancer Institute* 47:59–63, 1971.

Heinonen, O. P., D. Sloane, and S. Shapiro, eds., *Birth Defects and Drugs in Pregnancy.* Littleton, Mass.: Publishing Sciences Group, 1977, p. 246.

*Ibid.,* p. 363.

**p. 154** *Ibid.,* p. 492.

**p. 155** Dowty, B. J., J. L. Laester, and J. Storer, "The Transplacental Migration and Accumulation in Blood of Volatile Organic Constituents." *Pediatric Research* 10:696–701, 1976.

## CHAPTER SIX

**p. 157** Carmichael, I. H. E., and R. J. Berry, "Diagnostic X-rays in Late Pregnancy and in the Neonate." *Lancet,* February 14, 1976, pp. 351–52.

Kelley, K. M., *et al.,* "The Utilization and Efficacy of Pelvimetry." *American Journal of Roentgenology* 125:66–74, 1975.

**p. 158** Meyer, M., J. A. Tonascia, and T. Merz, "Long-term Effects of Prenatal X-ray on Development and Fertility of Human Females." *Biological and Environmental Effects of Low-level Radiation,* Vol. II, Vienna, Austria: International Atomic Energy Commission, 1976, pp. 273–84.

**p. 163** Silverman, C., and D. Hoffman, "Overview: Thyroid Tumor Risk from Radiation During Childhood." *Preventive Medicine* 4:100–5, 1975.

Hempelmann, L. H., and J. Grossman, "The Association of Illnesses with Abnormal Immunologic Features with Irradiation of the Thymic Gland in Infancy." *Radiation Research* 58:122–27, 1974.

Omran, A. R., R. E. Shore, R. A. Markoff, *et al.,* "Follow-up Study of Patients Treated by X-ray Epilation for Tinea Capitis: Psychiatric and Psychometric Evaluation. *American Journal of Public Health* 68:561–67, 1978.

**p. 165** Modan, B., *et al.,* "Radiation-induced Head and Neck Tumors." *Lancet,* February 23, 1974, pp. 277–79.

p. 166 Stewart, A., "Malignant Disease in Childhood and Diagnostic Radiation in Utero. *Lancet,* September 1, 1956, p. 447.

p. 167 Mole, R. H., "Late Effects of Diagnostic Radiation: Carcinogenesis." *British Medical Bulletin* 29:78–83, 1973.

Kelley, K. M., *et al.,* "The Utilization and Efficacy of Pelvimetry." *Op. cit.*

p. 169 Kato, H., "Mortality in Children Exposed to the A-bombs While in Utero." *American Journal of Epidemiology* 93:435–42, 1971.

Graham, S., M. L. Levin, A. M. Lilienfeld, *et al.,* "Preconception, Intrauterine and Postnatal Irradiation as Related to Leukemia." *National Cancer Institute Monograph No. 19,* pp. 347–71, 1966.

Bertell, R., "X-ray Exposure and Premature Aging." *Journal of Surgical Oncology* 9:379–91, 1977.

p. 170 Miller, R. W., and W. J. Blot, "Small Head Size After In-utero Exposure to Atomic Radiation." *Lancet,* October 14, 1972, pp. 784–87.

p. 172 Gillette, R., "Radiation Standards: The Last Word or At Least a Definitive One." *Science,* December 1, 1972, p. 967.

p. 177 Editorial: "Radiation and the Genetic Load." *Lancet,* October 25, 1975, pp. 803–4.

p. 178 Environmental Mutagen Society Committee 17, "Environmental Mutagenic Hazards." *Science,* February 14, 1975, pp. 503–14.

p. 179 *Biological Effects of Ionizing Radiation (BEIR Report).* Washington, D.C.: National Academy of Sciences, 1972, p. 48.

p. 180 Kato, H., W. J. Schull, and J. V. Neel, "A Cohort-type Study of Survival in the Children of Parents Exposed to Atomic Bombings." *American Journal of Human Genetics* 18:365, 1966.

Neel, J. V., H. Kato, and W. J. Schull, "Mortality in the Children of Atomic Bomb Survivors and Controls." *Genetics* 76:311–26, 1974.

p. 181 Luning, K. G., and A. G. Searle, "Estimates of the Genetic Risks from Ionizing Radiation. *Mutation Research* 12:291–304, 1971.

Frier-Maria, N., "Abortions, Chromosome Aberrations, and Radiation." *Serial Biology* 17:102–5, 1970.

Macht, S. H., and P. S. Lawrence, "Congenital Malformations from Exposure to Roentgen Radiation." *American Journal of Roentgenology* 73:442–66, 1955.

p. 182 Uchida, I. A., and E. J. Curtis: "A Possible Association Between Maternal Radiation and Mongolism." *Lancet,* October 14, 1961, pp. 848–50.

p. 183 *Biological Effects of Ionizing Radiation, op. cit.,* p. 69.

Alberman, E., *et al.,* "Parental Exposure to X-irradiation and Down's Syndrome." *Annals of Human Genetics* 36:195–208, 1972.

Alberman, E., *et al.,* "Parental Exposure to X-irradiation and Chromosome Constitution of Aborted Fetuses." *Annals of Human Genetics* 36:185–94, 1972.

p. 184 Stewart, A., J. Webb, and D. Hewitt, "A Survey of Childhood Malignancies." *British Medical Journal* 1:1495–1508, 1958.

p. 185 Twine, E. H., and E. J. Potchen, "A Dynamic Systems Analysis of

Defensive Medicine." M.S. Thesis, Massachusetts Institute of Technology, 1973. (not seen)

**p. 185** Eason, C., and B. Brooks, "Should Medical Radiation Exposures Be Recorded?" *American Journal of Public Health* 62:1189–93, 1972.

**p. 186** Caffey, J., in *Pediatric X-Ray Diagnosis*. Chicago: Yearbook Medical Publishers, 1972, p. *vii*.

Carmichael and Berry, "Diagnostic X-rays in Late Pregnancy and in the Neonate." *op. cit.*

**p. 188** Dobzhansky, T., *Mankind Evolving*. New Haven, Ct.: Yale University Press, 1962, p. 292.

## CHAPTER 7

**p. 190** "Sterility Linked to a Pesticide Sharpens Fear on Chemical Use," *New York Times,* September 11, 1977, p. 1.

**p. 191** Glass, R. I., R. N. Lyness, D. C. Mengle, *et al.,* "Sperm Count Depression in Pesticide Applicators Exposed to Dibromochloropropane." *American Journal of Epidemiology* 109:346–51, 1979.

Kapp, R., D. J. Picciano, and C. B. Jacobson, "Y-chromosomal Nondisjunction in Dibromochloropropane-exposed Workmen." *Mutation Research* 64:47–51, 1979.

**p. 194** Schroeder, H. A., and M. Mitchner, "Toxic Effects of Trace Elements on the Reproduction of Mice and Rats." *Archives of Environmental Health* 23:102–6, 1971.

**p. 195** "Rise in Birth Defects Laid to Job Hazards." *New York Times,* March 14, 1976, p. 1.

**p. 196** Hunt, V. R., *Occupational Health Problems of Pregnant Women*. Report to the Office of the HEW Secretary, 1975.

**p. 197** Pilger, John, "The Gook-Hunter." *New York Times,* April 26, 1979, p. A23.

**p. 198** *New York Times,* May 27, 1979, p. 42.

Whiteside, T., "A Reporter at Large (Seveso, Italy)." *New Yorker,* September 4, 1978, pp. 34–81.

**p. 199** "EPA, Citing Miscarraiges, Restricts Two Pesticides." *New York Times,* March 2, 1979, p. A10.

Braughman, R., M. Meselson, and P. O'Keefe, "Memorandum on Human Milk Monitoring; Preliminary Results for Twenty-Five Samples, March 1, 1977." (personal communication from Dr. Meselson)

**p. 200** Whiteside, T., "A Reporter at Large (The Pendulum and the Toxic Cloud)." *New Yorker,* July 25, 1977, p. 49.

**p. 202** Baltzer, B., A. Ericson, and A. Kallen, Letter: "Pregnancy Outcome Among Women Working in Swedish Hospitals." *New England Journal of Medicine* 300:627–28, 1979.

Whiteside, T., *New Yorker,* July 25, 1977, *op. cit.,* p. 51.

**p. 203** Shantz, S. L., D. A. Barsotti, and J. R. Allen, Abstract: "Toxicological

Effects Produced in Non-human Primates Chronically Exposed to 50 Parts per Trillion 2,3,7,8-Tetraclorodibenzo-p-dioxin (TCDD)." *Toxicology and Applied Pharmacology* 48:A-180, 1979.

p. 205 Lane, R., "The Spectre of Sterility." *Esquire,* April 11, 1978, pp. 30–33.

MacLeod, J., and Y. Wang, "Male Fertility Potential in Terms of Semen Quality: A Review of the Past, a Study of the Present." *Fertility-Sterility* 31:103–16, 1979.

p. 207 Brady, K., Y. Herrera, and H. Zenick, "Influence of Parental Lead Exposure on Subsequent Learning Ability of Offspring." *Pharmacology, Biochemistry and Behavior* 3:561–65, 1975.

Lancranjan, I., "Reproductive Ability of Workmen Occupationally Exposed to Lead." *Archives of Environmental Health* 30:396–401, 1975.

p. 210 Erickson, J. D., W. M. Cochran, and C. E. Anderson, "Birth Defects and Parental Occupation: Preliminary Results from Metropolitan Atlanta." In press.

Hricko, A., "Today's Job Hazard vs. Tomorrow's Baby." *Los Angeles Times,* May 28, 1977, Part II, p. 7.

p. 211 Quimby, K. L., *et al.,* "Enduring Learning Deficits and Cerebral Synaptic Malformation from Exposure to 10 Parts of Halothane per Million." *Science,* August 16, 1974, pp. 625–27.

p. 213 *Michigan Health Statistics,* 1961–1977, and unpublished data. Lansing, Mich.: Office of Vital and Health Statistics, Michigan Department of Public Health.

Wharton, D., R. M. Krauss, S. Marshall, *et al.,* "Infertility in Male Pesticide Workers." *Lancet,* December 17, 1977, pp. 1259–61.

## CHAPTER EIGHT

p. 214 "The Susceptibility of the Fetus and Child to Chemical Pollutants." *Pediatrics* (Suppl.) 53, 1974.

p. 215 Hillman, L. S., *et al.,* "Identification and Measurement of Plasticizer in Neonatal Tissues After Umbilical Catheters and Blood Products," *New England Journal of Medicine* 292:381–86.

"Routine Fetal Monitoring Is Termed Costly and Unsafe." *New York Times,* January 2, 1979, p. C3.

Paul, R. H., J. R. Huey, and C. F. Yaeger, "Clinical Fetal Monitoring." *Postgraduate Medicine* 61:160–66, 1977.

p. 216 Chalmers, I., Commentary: "British Debate on Obstetric Practice." *Pediatrics* 58:308–12, 1976.

p. 218 Emanuel, I., "Problems of Outcome of Pregnancy." *Birth Defects: Risks and Consequences,* S. Kelly, ed. Albany, N.Y.: Academic Press, 1974, pp. 119–34.

Brackbill, Y., and H. Berendes, Letter: "Dangers of Diethylstilbestrol." *Lancet,* September 2, 1978, p. 520.

p. 219 Goldenberg, R. L., and K. Nelson, "Iatrogenic Respiratory Distress Syndrome." *American Journal of Obstetrics and Gynecology* 123:617–20, 1975.

p. 221 Campbell, N., D. Harvery, and A. P. Norman, "Increased Frequency of

Neonatal Jaundice in a Maternity Hospital." *British Medical Journal* 2:548–52, 1975.

**p. 222** Sims, D. G., and G. A. Neligan, "Factors Affecting the Increasing Incidence of Severe Non-haemolytic Neonatal Jaundice." *British Journal of Obstetrics and Gynecology* 82:863–67, 1975.

Scheidt, P. C., E. D. Mellitts, J. B. Hardy, *et al.*, "Toxicity to Bilirubin in Neonates." *Journal of Pediatrics* 91:292–97, 1977.

**p. 223** Dunn, P. M., "Obstetric Delivery Today: For Better or Worse?" *Lancet*, April 10, 1976, pp. 790–93.

**p. 224** Kroener, W. F., Jr., quoted in discussion following "Changing Trends in Cesarean Section." *American Journal of Obstetrics and Gynecology* 125:798–804, 1976.

**p. 225** Edington, P. T., J. Sibanda, and R. W. Beard: "Influence on Clinical Practice of Routine Intrapartum Fetal Monitoring," *British Medical Journal*, Vol. 3, pp. 341–343.

**p. 227** Klaus, M. H., R. Jerauld, N. C. Kreger, *et al.*, "Maternal Attachment: Importance of the First Post-partum Days." *New England Journal of Medicine* 286:460–63, 1972.

**p. 229** Benson, R. C., H. Berendes, and W. Weiss, "Fetal Compromise During Elective Cesarean Section." *American Journal of Obstetrics and Gynecology* 105:579–96, 1969.

**p. 230** Brackbill, Y., and S. Broman, Draft: "Obstetrical Medication and Development in the First Year of Life." Bethesda, Md.: National Institute of Neurological and Communicative Disorders and Stroke, January 1979.

**p. 235** Hughey, M. J., T. H. McElin, and T. Young, "Maternal and Fetal Outcome of Lamaze-prepared Patients." *Obstetrics and Gynecology* 51:643–47, 1978.

**p. 236** Dr. Kaminetzky quoted in *Medical World News*, July 24, 1978.

**p. 237** Summaries, in *Prevention of Embryonic, Fetal and Perinatal Disease*, R. L. Brent and M. I. Harris, eds. Bethesda, Md.: National Institutes of Health (HEW Publication No. NIH-76-853), 1976.

Wegman, M. E., "Annual Summary of Vital Statistics." *Pediatrics* 62:947–54, 1978.

**p. 238** Pomerance, J. J., C. T. Ukrainski, T. Ukra, *et al*, "Cost of Living for Infants Weighing 1,000 Grams or Less at Birth." *Pediatrics* 61:908–10, 1978.

**p. 239** Browne, H. E., and G. Isaacs, "The Frontier Nursing Service: The Primary Care Nurse in the Community Hospital." *American Journal of Obstetrics and Gynecology* 124:14–17, 1976.

**p. 242** Epstein, S., *The Politics of Cancer*. San Francisco: Sierra Club Books, 1978, p. 441.

**p. 243** Terrill, J. G., "Cost-benefit Estimates for the Major Sources of Radiation Exposure." *American Journal of Public Health* 62:1008–13, 1972.

**p. 246** Judge Harvey Quoted in the *New York Times*, May 27, 1979, p. 42.

**p. 247** Sunstein, E., *A Different Face*. New York: Harper & Row, 1975, p. 257.

# SELECTED READINGS

*The following is a list of book chapters and articles, in both the scientific and general press, which are helpful overviews of some of the major subjects discussed in the text.*

"Birth Defects and Their Environmental Causes," *Medical World News*, January 21, 1971, p. 47.

Bibbo, M., W. B. Gill, F. Azizi *et al.*, "Follow-up Study of Male and Female Offspring of DES-Exposed Mothers." *Journal of Obstetrics and Gynecology*, 49:1–8, 1977.

Brent, R. L., "Litigation Produced Pain, Disease and Suffering: An Experience with Congenital Malformation Lawsuits." *Teratology* 16:1–14, 1977.

Brodeur, P., "The Genetic Time-Bomb." In: *The Zapping of America*. New York: W. W. Norton and Company, 1977, pp. 132–152.

Burnham, D., "Rise in Birth Defects Laid to Job Hazards." *New York Times*, March 14, 1976, p. 1.

Chisolm, J. J., Jr, "Fouling One's Own Nest." *Pediatrics* 62: 614–17, 1978.

Dunn, P., "Obstetric Delivery Today: For Better or Worse?" *Lancet*, April 10, 1976, pp. 790–93.

Kalota, G. B., Behavioral Teratology: Birth Defects of the Mind. *Science*, November 17, 1978, pp. 732–4.

Kane, D. N., "The Air Children Breathe." *The Nation*, August 28, 1976, p. 143.

Kelley, K. M., *et al.*, "The Utilization and Efficacy of Pelvimetry." *American Journal of Roentgenology* 125:66–75, 1975.

Legator, M., and S. Rinkus, "The Chemical Environment and Mutagenesis." *Proceedings of a Conference on Women and the Workplace*, Washington, D.C.: The Society for Occupational and Environmental Health, 1977, pp. 5–20.

Meyer, M. B., and J. A. Tonascia, "Maternal Smoking, Pregnancy Complications and Perinatal Mortality." *American Journal of Obstetrics and Gynecology* 128:494–502, 1977.

Maugh, T. H. II, "Chemical Carcinogens: The Scientific Basis for Regulation." *Science*, September 29, 1978, pp. 1200–5.

Rice, J., "An Overview of Transplacental Carcinogenesis." *Teratology* 8:113–26, 1973.

Ross, D., and S. A. Ross: "Etiological Factors in Hyperactivity—Environmental Factors." In: *Hyperactivity: Research, Theory and Action*. New York: Wiley, 1976, pp. 81–94.

Spyker, J., "Assessing the Impact of Low Level Chemicals on Development: Behavioral and Latent Effects." *Federation Proceedings* 34:1835–44, 1975.

Whiteside, T., "A Reporter at Large (The Pendulum and the Toxic Cloud)." *New Yorker*, July 25, 1977.

# INDEX